Technicians of the Finite

Contributions in Medical History
Series Editor: John Burnham

Women & Men Midwives
Medicine, Morality, and Misogyny in Early America
Jane B. Donegan

American Midwives 1860 to the Present
Judy Barrett Litoff

Speech and Speech Disorders in Western Thought
Before 1600
Ynez Violé O'Neill

Sex, Diet, and Debility in Jacksonian America:
Sylvester Graham and Health Reform
Stephen Nissenbaum

Shock, Physiological Surgery, and George Washington Crile:
Medical Innovation in the Progressive Era
Peter C. English

Professionalizing Modern Medicine: Paris Surgeons and
Medical Science and Institutions in the 18th Century
Toby Gelfand

Medicine and Its Technology: An Introduction
to the History of Medical Instrumentation
Audrey B. Davis

In Her Own Words: Oral Histories of Women Physicians
*Regina Markell Morantz, Cynthia Stodola Pomerleau, and
Carol Hansen Fenichel, editors*

Technicians of the Finite

THE RISE AND DECLINE OF
THE SCHIZOPHRENIC IN
AMERICAN THOUGHT
1840-1960

S. P. Fullinwider

CONTRIBUTIONS IN MEDICAL HISTORY NUMBER 9

Greenwood Press

WESTPORT, CONNECTICUT · LONDON, ENGLAND

Library of Congress Cataloging in Publication Data

Fullinwider, S. P.
    Technicians of the finite.

    (Contributions in medical history, ISSN 0147-1058;
no. 9)
    Bibliography: p.
    Includes index.
    1. Psychiatry—Philosophy—United States—History.
2. Schizophrenia—Philosophy—United States—History.
3. Social Psychiatry—United States—History.   I. Title.
II. Series.   [DNLM: 1. Schizophrenia—History—United
States.   2. Psychiatry—History—United States.   WM 11
AA1 F9t]
RC339.A1F84   616.8'982   81-23771
ISBN 0-313-23021-8   (lib.bdg.)   AACR2

Library of Congress Catalog Card Number: 81-23771
ISBN: 0-313-23021-8
ISSN: 0147-1058

First published in 1982

Greenwood Press
A division of Congressional Information Service, Inc.
88 Post Road West
Westport, Connecticut 06881

Printed in the United States of America

10 9 8 7 6 5 4 3 2 1

To Mr. Peters

CONTENTS

ACKNOWLEDGMENTS

My debt to those who helped along the way is heartfelt: to Mary Kaczmarek for struggling to make these pages readable; to Richard Barlow, William Williams, John Stone, Garth Blackham, and Daniel Blackwood, for their critical readings of portions of the manuscript; to series editor John Burnham, for his all-important critique; to the Rockefeller Foundation, for a 1975–1976 Humanities Fellowship; to Robert Henning, for listening to my ideas when we were both in a condition to appreciate them.

Technicians of the Finite

INTRODUCTION

In recent years several critics of the modern understanding and treatment of mental illness (Thomas Szasz, Michel Foucault, Erving Goffman) have suggested that we look less at the patients and more at the social and ideological processes that have given rise to our conceptions and perceptions of the mentally ill. *Technicians of the Finite* is an attempt to throw some new light on the concept of schizophrenia as it began to emerge in nineteenth-century America and as it dominated the psychiatric landscape of the twentieth century. In turn, by using the concept of schizophrenia as an example of modern thought processes, I hope to bring some insight to the way certain underlying social processes have acted to structure twentieth-century thought. My approach is historical, though I attempt no comprehensive history of the idea or treatment of schizophrenia. My mode of analysis will be that of the sociology of ideas; but at no point will I attempt to deny the fact of mental illness or attempt to comment on its nature.

At times I will focus on broad theoretical movements within American psychiatry—the "moral insanity" debate of the nineteenth century (chapter 1), the Americanization of Freudian theory in the 1920s and 1930s (chapter 5), and the shift to systems theory in the 1960s (chapter 8). At other times the focus will be on the interaction between psychiatrist and patient—a classic case in multiple personality at the turn of the century (chapter 2) and post-World War II attempts to deal with schizophrenics (chapter 6). At still other times it will be necessary to range beyond psychiatry proper, into the formative psychologies of William James (chapter 3) and G. Stanley Hall (chapter 4) and into certain decisive developments in brain neurology.

The shifts in focus will be used to develop two unifying themes, one that is strictly historical, the other in the sociology of ideas. The

3

historical unity lies in tracing for the first time the development of the "higher-lower doctrine": the belief that the human nervous system is so structured that within each of us there is a higher, rational level and a lower, irrational level. In American neuropsychiatric circles, from the late nineteenth century until the mid-twentieth century, it was universally believed that insanity involved the weakening of the higher nervous levels and the dominance of the lower. The higher-lower doctrine gave technical neurophysiological support to a series of ideas—one might say a mythology—crucial to American psychiatry. The ideas about the "lower man"—that he was a *savage* and that he was a *machine* living in a *dream*—were formulated late in the nineteenth century and gave shape to much that was to come later. It is the strictly historical task of *Technicians of the Finite* to trace the development of these ideas as they structured the definition and treatment of schizophrenia, as they influenced the way Freudian theory was received and reformulated in America, and as they functioned in the development of a mental health ideology.

The ideas about the lower of the higher-lower doctrine were also metaphors, however; metaphors that described what psychiatrists saw and felt when face-to-face with certain forms of mental illness. For this reason it is important to delve into the chemistry of the doctor-patient relationship in such cases. It is at this point that the sociology of ideas approach becomes relevant. The problem is to arrive at an understanding of the socio-psychological roots of the several metaphors. It therefore becomes necessary to place the doctor-patient relationship in its social and intellectual environment.

It will be seen that certain sorts of people—those the profession learned to call schizophrenics—place an almost unbearable perceptual strain on the psychiatrist. As the doctor confronts the patient he feels his world break apart. He begins to lose perceptual control over his environment. We discover that the words used by the psychiatrist to describe the schizophrenic patient—"savage," "dream," "machine" —were in reality metaphors for his own perceptual disorganization. We conclude that his medical attempts to restructure the patient were infused with a struggle to regain control for himself.

We are forced to ask ourselves—and this is the goal of the sociology of ideas approach—what in American life provides us with our fundamental perceptual structuring of our world and how it is that certain people or certain sorts of behavior have the power to threaten that structure. Since the metaphors will be our main gateways, it will be well to take a closer look at them now and to let them introduce certain theoretical considerations.

MACHINE

All people of all times have used shared conceptual mappings of their worlds. A mapping guides perception, giving what is seen its intelligibility, if not its meaning. But because the world is infinite in its complexity and all mappings are limited, events will come to the attention that seem to violate any given mapping because they make no sense within its context. These events are part of the world's overflow; they seep through the edges and the seams of the mapping, but because they can be thought of as what the mapping leaves behind, I will call them the "residue." Such events, when attended to, will be unpredictable and will therefore seem random. No doubt all cultures develop residual categories to make sense out of these sorts of events. A religious age that emphasizes a rational God—the age of the American Puritans, for example—might (as the Puritans did) describe such a category in terms of the demonic.

In early and mid-nineteenth-century America, when neuropsychiatry got its start, the reigning conceptual mapping within the sciences was what has been called "doxological" science, featuring as its base assumption a world that reflects God's design. The ruling assumption was that every happening and each phenomenon is a means toward a divinely appointed end. The doxological mapping emphasized a means-end causality in which the means (for example, the stomach) is linked through design to its end (digestion). This approach was not challenged by nineteenth-century American scientists until Darwinian theory made its impact. After that, as scientific naturalism with its mechanistic assumptions began to gain ground, American neuro-psychiatry began its century-long stand as a rear guard action in behalf of the doxological mapping in the human sciences. It was the conception of the insane person as a machine that enabled neuro-psychiatry to assume this role.

Certain sorts of behavior, for example the brutal murder that seemed to proceed from no recognizable motive, stood in direct violation of the means-end mapping. It was nothing new when nineteenth-century physicians for the mentally ill turned to somatic (for example, brain disease) explanations for this sort of behavior; the somatic explanation went back at least to Hippocrates and the ancient Greeks. What was new was the way the somatic explanation was used. The insane person was now said to have become an automaton, or machine, who has lost his higher (human) faculties and his selfhood. The implication of this assertion, which American psychiatry was quick to take up and defend, was that the normal person has a spiritual element (the conscious ego) which lifts him above the realm of mechanism and determinism. European psychiatry, and in particular Freud, did not make this assumption, and therein lies the great difference. For the Americans, assuming as they did that to be normal is to have this spiritual element, normality became the great desideratum. To be fully human, one had to be normal.

SAVAGE

The demonic, which plagued the Puritans, had been dormant for well over a hundred years when it reemerged in a new guise, as the "savage of moral insanity." Here again causality was reestablished in cases that otherwise seemed random. A savage personality was envisioned as lying hidden within, one which could suddenly, without warning, take over control of the body and sometimes the consciousness of the insane. The machine metaphor actually came into being as a reaction against the new demonic by opponents of the theory of moral insanity, but the two, savage and machine, were categories for the residual within the context of the doxological mapping. Both were metaphors for the loss of perceptual control over the offender; both were, therefore, metaphors for the uncontrolled.

Both metaphors—savage and machine—were destined by the late nineteenth century to be brought together as twin elements of the lower in the higher-lower doctrine. In either case the patient was perceived to have lost his true selfhood. This selfhood was understood to be regained if and when the patient reestablished control over the savage within. From one point of view, selfhood was considered regained when the psychiatrist reestablished perceptual control.

Another way of saying this is to describe the psychiatrist's notion of the patient's "real self" as his term for his own perceptual control over the patient: when the patient responded as desired, in a way to establish the psychiatrist's security in the patient's presence, the patient was considered to have a real self and to be sane.

DREAM

It is with the dream metaphor that we enter into the real complexity of our subject, and it is here that we come to grips with psychiatry's great contribution to twentieth-century thought, the notion of the unconscious. The unconscious, as American psychiatry came to understand it, embodied the savage and the machine. But it was itself the embodiment of the dream metaphor. With one small exception, I have not taken the liberty to make any assumptions about the development of the concept of the unconscious in Europe. That would be a subject for a different book. I wish only to show what became of the notion when the Americans adopted it.

If the savage and the machine were metaphorical statements for the sense of the uncaused and the sense of lost perceptual control, the dream was a metaphor for the perceptual disorganization itself, the disorganization into which the psychiatrist was plunged when facing the uncaused. Unravelling the dream metaphor gets us directly into the dynamics of the psychiatrist-patient relation. The psychiatrist learned to react to his perceptual disorganization by attempting to restructure his world, in the first place by assigning a cause (machine, savage) to the patient's behavior, but in the long run by attempting to restore the patient's real self.

But the dream situation involved the doctor-patient relation in a complex process not yet outlined. The psychiatrist's own selfhood was at stake in his perceptual disorientation. I rely on George Herbert Mead's theory of the dynamics of self-construction to guide us in following the sequence of events that were involved. According to Mead, one's own (for example, the psychiatrist's) self is achieved through, and structured by, the anticipated responses to be made to him by significant others (for example, the patient). Mead designated this sense of selfhood the "me." He argued that when the other's responses violate one's anticipations, the "me" begins to waver and fail, ultimately giving way to an "I," a situation of unreflective, and therefore impulsive, behavior. The "me" situation exists when one is able to anticipate and thus respond to one's *own* responses by taking the point of view of the other toward oneself. The "I" (the state of disorientation) emerges and replaces the "me" when one is no longer able to anticipate one's own behavior owing to the fact that it has become impossible to take the other's point of view. At that point one's own behavior becomes erratic and unpredictable. To sum up Mead's argument, we might say that one achieves a self when one can anticipate the other's responses; conversely, one's self is threatened when the other ceases to respond predictably. It becomes clear from Mead's argument that the psychiatrist's "me" is at stake as he struggles for perceptual control over the patient.

For us, the dream metaphor must indicate not only the psychiatrist's loss of perceptual control over the patient, but over himself as well. With the sensed loss of self-control, the inability, that is, to anticipate his own responses, the psychiatrist feels the savage rise within himself. The machine metaphor also has a role here. It represents the psychiatrist's growing tendency, when interacting with the schizophrenic patient, to become an object to himself, an object in the sense of being alien and uncontrolled. Ultimately, it is the attempt to break out of his own dreamlike experience with its threat from the savage within that explains why the psychiatrist works to objectify the patient.

THE DIALECTIC OF OBJECTIFICATION

By "objectification" I mean the attempt to restore conceptual mapping when it has been violated. As I use the term, it involves most centrally the process of forming a residual category of events that do not fit the mapping and then bringing this residual category back into the mapping. Since the mapping defines the public reality, events which violate a mapping are considered private. Objectification is the process by which the private is made public. The process of objectification pertains specifically to the mechanistic mapping in which the public reality was said to be "objective."

Objectification was pursued in the attempt to regain perceptual control. However, the interrelated processes of objectifying the patient and self-objectification described above often promoted a downward spiral into increasing perceptual disorganization. There appears, indeed, to have been a dynamic involved in the process, a dynamic I will identify as a "dialectic of objectification," where each step taken toward objectification caused a further degree of perceptual disorganization and where each new degree of perceptual disorganization precipitated a new step toward further objectification. The dialectic of objectification, as it occurred in the doctor-patient relation, will be more fully developed in chapter 2. Here it is enough to add that my working definition of schizophrenia will be that relation between psychiatrist and patient where the dialectic is irreversibly present.

THE NON-CARTESIAN DUALISM

As it unfolded in the doctor-patient relation, the dialectic of objectification tended to break down that line between subject and object that supported the Cartesian dualism and the conceptual mappings dependent on that dualism. The line was violated when the doctor became object to himself as a result of the dialectical process. In face of the patient's unpredictability, the doctor's own behavior became first tentative, then unpredictable to himself; a dialectic of self-objectification ensued, drawing the doctor step-by-step into further degrees of self-objectification. The doctor entered the domain of the non-Cartesian dualism: a dualism of two side-by-side worlds. In one world everything, including the doctor's most private responses, became object; in the other world everything was dreamlike, insubstantial, and random, due to the doctor's perceptual disorientation.

For the psychiatrists of the late nineteenth century, the line that establishes the distinction between subject and object was being threatened from another direction; that is, from the steps being made by scientific naturalism toward mechanistic theory. Neurophysiology, for example, tried to keep a distinction between sensory excitation (objective) and sensation (subjective), but reflex-arc theory did not need that distinction. In it everything was reduced to objective data.

In America it was William James, a trained physiologist, who first followed the lead of reflex-arc theory to its ultimate conclusion. In his *Principles of Psychology* (1890), he found that he could reduce each and every "subjective" event to objective data. He found that the innermost "I," the self-observing self, could be reduced to muscular tensions in the neck, glottis, and backward-rolling eyeballs. He devoted a chapter to that demonstration, but in the following chapter he turned the tables, and reinterpreting all so-called objective data as subjective events, he portrayed a dreamlike world defined by an infinity of ever-changing events, the stream of consciousness. In two back-to-back chapters, James had portrayed the non-Cartesian dualism in a way that could not be dismissed thereafter. It was the outcome that necessarily followed when the Cartesian line between subject and object was dissolved by advancing mechanism.

But James's career shows that the pressures leading toward the non-Cartesian dualism were social as well as theoretical. He experienced his world and his selfhood dissolving before he described it in the *Principles*. In chapter 3, I will take a very close look at his experience. The evidence will suggest that in this regard we look at James as a representative figure of the genteel caste.

THE PROFESSIONALIZATION OF THE GENTEEL

To gain a fuller understanding of the social base of the doctor-patient relationship that began to emerge at the start of this century, it is useful to think in terms of the rise of the modern professional and, as a theoretical point of departure, the social-theoretic work done by the Frankfurt School, the school of Theodor Adorno, Max Horkheimer, and Herbert Marcuse. Their subject matter has been the historically simultaneous rise of the "commodity" and the "object" to dominance in our conceptual mapping of the world. An illustration will capture the spirit of their message: The ancient (c. 1300 A.D.) French *domus*, which signified home, family, and relatedness of the individual to his community and to the sacred past, becomes transformed in our time into the marketable commodity, the *house*. It is not simply that in modern society families move with great ease from locality to locality and from house to house. It is also that our angle of vision strips away from a dwelling all those "subjective" values that defined the *domus* and narrows to the single dimension of "market value." The house, as we know it, is a commodity and became that partly because the modern public reality, as defined by science, consists solely of objects. The ancient French *domus* stood at the center of the individual's sacred space, but there is now no longer room in the public reality for the sacred.

The genteel caste of late-nineteenth-century America was one of the last groups to cling to the sort of sacred space once defined by the *domus*. One thinks of Horatio Alger's young men valiantly trying to bring Christian goodness to the capitalist marketplace, of William Dean Howells' sense of invasion as he watched the Irish bring their alien ways to Boston and Cambridge, and of Mark Twain's sense of loss when he rediscovered the Mississippi from the vantage point of scientific naturalism. These examples might be multiplied endlessly. The genteel were to some extent still involved in the sort of ceremonial life that marks traditional cultures and that binds what we moderns have learned to think of as subjective feelings to the life of a group and to a place, making group and place sacred. Generally speaking, it was from the genteel that American neuropsychiatry emerged in the twentieth century. Its lingering commitment to the doxological mapping was its final expression of its sense of the sacred.

The work done by the Frankfurt School gives us a first step toward understanding the correlation between capitalist controls over the individual and the methods of science. In the everlasting balancing act between institutional controls and individual self-expression, the commodity and the object hold the intermediate position of self-imposed controls. Conceptual mappings are self-imposed controls in this sense: one imposes his mapping and then makes his behavior conform to it. The commodity is central to capitalist mapping, and the commodity became possible because it shared the property of being an object. In their role as mercantile capitalists, the genteel had thrived under this sort of mapping for nearly two centuries. Commodities, dissociated from "subjective" values, could be traded at will, based only on their exchange value. But as labor and labor time became defined by exchange value, one's tendency to get sucked into the abstract realm of exchange value (as a commodity, therefore as an object), increased. After the Civil War, when the mercantile capitalist class was being brushed aside by the new industrial class of capitalists and as the genteel consequently began to enter the market looking for jobs, the tendency reached crisis proportions. Ceremony and customs had once fashioned for the genteel a sacred space separate from the marketplace. That was no longer possible, but a modified doxological mapping was.

MENTAL HEALTH LIBERALISM

The confluence of three sorts of events — the doctor-patient dialectic, scientific naturalism, the genteel's shifting social circumstances — joined to threaten the security of the Cartesian dualism and, therefore, to undermine the foundations of the nineteenth-century mappings. G. Stanley Hall's two volume *Adolescence* (1905) was the central document in resolving the crisis. The non-Cartesian dualism was said by Hall to characterize a lower order of consciousness — the consciousness of the adolescent, of mass man, and of the schizophrenic. Through "emergence" the normal individual can arrive at a higher consciousness, the shared consciousness exercised by community in which the individual (non-Cartesian) consciousness somehow disappears. Hall made the higher consciousness a realm of perfect order. Other theorists, first the New Realist philosophers, later the system theorists, would define that order in terms of mathematical logic or the artificial intelligence of the information-processing machine. Hall gave American neuropsychiatry the foundation for a new ideology, which I will call "mental health liberalism." Psychiatric therapy would bring the patient out of the lower order of consciousness into the higher consciousness of community, that is to say, into the realm of perceptual clarity.

THE DIALECTIC IN HISTORY

As one looks over the field, one begins to see a certain rhythm: the threat to the conceptual mapping, mounting pressure toward defending that mapping, pressure that results in building up a residual category to the point at which the residue overwhelms the mapping and a conceptual reorganization takes place.

This process took place in the period from 1890 to 1900, resulting in mental health liberalism and the Americanization of Freudian theory to conform to that ideology; it took place once again in the 1950s to 1960s with the collapse of the higher-lower doctrine in both psychiatry and neurophysiology. Each collapse and reorganization brought a shift in theory to a level of abstraction one step further removed from experience. In the earlier crisis the individual was replaced by the "community" as the functioning unit. In the later period, the material world was replaced by information. In each case the older conceptual mapping fell prey to the infinite seeping through and overlapping its boundaries.

1

THE NINETEENTH-CENTURY BACKGROUND

The nineteenth century defined insanity; the twentieth century worked out the implications of that effort. In America the roots of men's reactions to the mentally ill go back somewhat ambivalently to the seventeenth-century rural community's sometimes easy toleration of deviance and the Puritan's quickness to see manifestations of God's wrath. The nineteenth century did not give us the medical approach—the belief that mental illness has natural causes—the Greeks gave us that, but it enshrined science and gave us the asylum movement. It gave us as our first psychiatrists the asylum physicians of the Jacksonian era.

The nineteenth century has been described as revolutionary in its treatment of the insane in refusing to treat them as less than human.[1] Historians say that its reformers refused to believe that mental illness touches the immortal soul. I will not deny that this is what they said and believed, only that this is not what they *perceived*. They *saw* the individual's selfhood melt away before their eyes. It was this perception that was destined to define insanity for the twentieth century.

Certain historians suggest that the asylum movement was a response to growing faith in science and progress and to developing humanitarian feeling—all products of the Enlightenment.[2] Some argue that the nineteenth century rejected the older view that insanity is a choice for the irrational over the rational and saw it instead as the alienation of the individual from nature.[3] These beliefs were indeed much on the lips of Jacksonian era physicians. The asylums were supposed to put the sick into healing contact with nature. The problem with this interpretation is that the physicians' view of nature was becoming changed to that of the mechanistic side of Newtonian

14

science, a world consisting of mere objects. And what the physicians perceived in their patients was undergoing this same transformation.

Yet another approach to the asylum movement sees it manifesting the end of a dialogue between "Reason" and "Unreason."[4] Michel Foucault tells us that seventeenth- and eighteenth-century rationalism in effect cordoned off the "irrational" into asylums to avoid learning from it. This approach makes a great deal of sense if we remove the capitals from "reason" and "unreason." The insane were to become like the shark-infested and cannibalistic ocean depths of Melville's classic, the mirror revealing, to those who dared look, the animalistic and nonhuman aspects of human society. But few dared look. The rest, by attributing nonhumanity to the fact of insanity, were able to disguise what they were seeing and to deny it in themselves.

Historians have emphasized that the asylum physicians of the day believed that lust after wealth and rank was leading many into disappointment and insanity.[5] What the historians have not noticed is the grave concern with which the physicians viewed the several forms of extreme inner-directedness confronting them in American society. They saw social climbing all about them where, as they thought, people once had been content with their lives; they saw men's minds imprisoned in desperate reformist fantasies; they saw people leaping into a subjective pit of religious fanaticism, withdrawing from the contact the physicians believed one achieves with God through the healthy unity with nature.[6]

The physicians were but reporting the results of a century or more of political and economic factionalism in American life, which had the cumulative effect of undermining tradition and traditional authority figures and institutions.[7] Outside the circles of the rich, the tendency was toward uprootedness, movement, and the conjugal family and away from community ties and the extended family.[8] The physicians' complaints registered what they themselves were experiencing: among large sectors of the population the individual's subjective life was ceasing to be public property. It was becoming private and, to the observer, enigmatic.

What was new in the Jacksonian-era medical mind was not any specific notions about the etiology of insanity. The idea of the "insane impulse" that so excited the medical imagination, for example, was a concern to English physician Thomas Arnold back in 1782. "I call that impulsive insanity," he wrote, "in which the patient is impelled to do, or say, what is highly imprudent, improper, unreasonable, impertinent, ridiculous, or absurd, without sufficient, with very slight, or with no apparent cause."[9] What was new in the 1830s was the beginning of an unconscious shift away from an essentialist perspective toward the insane. Isaac Ray of Butler Hospital, Rhode Island, a leading advocate of the doctrine of "moral insanity," found himself denying that his somatic analysis of insanity implicated the immortal soul in the disease process. But all the while that he held steadfast to his belief in the soul, he erratically skidded toward a perception of the insane as lacking selves. The only sure indication of insanity, he insisted, is the individual's sudden change of character when there is no observable cause to otherwise account for it. The individual must always be compared with himself; if he is not his old self, then he is insane.[10] John Gray of Utica Asylum in New York, at mid-century one of the younger generation of asylum superintendents and a leader of the assault against the doctrine of moral insanity, tirelessly and unkindly indicted Ray for abandoning the immortal soul. But in adopting the English reflex-arc explanation of human behavior, Gray went much further than his adversary in seeing insanity as the loss of selfhood. Gray's insane person was a simple reflex-arc machine, totally lacking any kind of human essence.

Few American physicians in the nineteenth century openly tried to discredit the soul. They simply made the matter moot. The question of selfhood took over. The self was something they could see — or thought they could — and in the insane they could see it disappear — or thought they could. By the end of the century their textbooks assumed the degeneracy and savagery of the paranoid, the "moral idiot," and the epileptic — assumptions made popular in Europe by the Italian Cesare Lombroso and the Germans R. von Krafft-Ebing and Max Nordau.[11] Whatever they might say about the immortal soul, the Americans were on their way towards perceiving the insane in nonhuman terms.

To gauge the real shift in nineteenth-century attitudes toward the mentally ill, we must go back to a generation before the first group of asylum superintendents, back to the generation that included Benjamin Rush and his European contemporaries. Rush and certain of the

Europeans, Philippe Pinel and Jean Esquirol, for instance, brought patience, humanitarian understanding, and faith in science to their dealings with the insane. These things they passed on to their successors. What they were unable to pass on was their firm belief that the insane individual was still very much himself.

Rush's generation held that the insane individual was simply exaggerating his normal character and temperament. He was too much himself, so to speak: if normally easy to anger, he was insanely angry; if normally susceptible to sadness and depression, he was insanely sad and depressed. Mania and melancholia, the chief disease categories, were ancient names reflecting the presumed reigning emotions. Esquirol went so far as to write a treatise (*Des Passions*, 1805) to prove that insanity is defined by its ruling emotion. For Rush mania was "madness," or "phrenetic disposition," or "rage." For Pinel it was "an undue indulgence of the angry passions." For Esquirol it was "an excess of prolonged anger. . . . "[12] A bit later, John Conolly in England described insanity as the result of "an exaggeration of common passions and emotions. . . . "[13] None of these men thought that insanity meant a change in character, much less a loss of self.

It took time to evolve the idea that the civilized self masks an insane savage within. Those who chose to follow the English physician-physiologist James Cowles Prichard in embracing the concept of moral insanity took the first major step. Writing in 1835, Prichard was incensed by court convictions of the obviously insane. Courts listened to the plea of insanity only where intellectual derangement could be amply demonstrated. The plea of an insane impulse offered no escape. Prichard urged that many insane persons reason correctly and are even horrified by their actions; the governing principle should be that an antisocial act is insane when it is foreign to the individual's nature. So taught Prichard, reversing the accepted rationale.

Contemporary medical literature was full of chilling tales: brutal murders of infants, incredible sexual acts, and combinations of sexual bestiality and cannibalism. Many of the perpetrators seemed astonished at themselves. Others, far more repellent to Prichard, seemed indifferent, and impersonal. In contemplating these things, Prichard found himself pushed to use words strange to the ears of science. He wrote of "other instances in which malignity has a deeper dye. The individual [acts] as if actually possessed by the demon of evil. . . . " Here was the first hint of an alien force, an invasion from outside.[14]

In a sense, Prichard was returning to the notion of madness widespread during the waning years of the Middle Ages, a period before the seventeenth and eighteenth centuries — the Age of Reason — defined the irrational as mere absence of reason. According to historian George Rosen, people of the fifteenth and sixteenth centuries thought madness, the irrational, to have an independent existence, to be a force in itself, and to constitute an invasion from without. By the 1830s the impact of English and French empiricist medicine and Lockean-based psychology had established the doctrine that mental illness usually results from some sort of somatic disorder. A disordered brain was thought to affect perceptions. Delusions, hallucinations, and wrong associations of ideas were the result of an inability to process sensory input from the outside world. Pinel, Esquirol, and others, including Rush, recognized a disorder that did not involve intellectual derangement and therefore could not be explained as a disordering of the senses.[15] It was this sort of disorder Prichard was trying to explain and to use as an explanation for certain horrible acts. Prichard's contribution was to revive the notion of an alien force.

In 1856 asylum superintendent J. J. Quinn was fascinated by the case of the Cincinnati, Ohio, murderer, Nancy Farrer. Acting as housekeeper for several families in succession, Miss Farrer left in her wake a disturbing number of corpses. She liked to flavor her cooking with arsenic. What stunned the authorities and sent Nancy to the asylum was that she had no apparent motive. Quinn commented: "During the eight months she has been under the writer's observation, the closest scrutiny has been unable to detect the least evidence of mental weakness — or intellectual or moral impairment . . . and yet it is difficult to reconcile the poisoning of so many innocent and harmless persons with her amiable and kind-hearted, and affectionate disposition, without supposing the presence, at the time, of an irrational motive or insane impulse."[16]

Quinn was saying, in effect, that you can't always trust your senses. The Miss Farrer he saw before him was somehow not real. In showing no sign of criminality or disease, her personality seemed to disclose the presence of disease the way a mask discloses the face it is hiding. It was her very personableness that made her crime, by contrast, so impersonal. Had she been outwardly cold and ruthless, she would surely have been imprisoned for life. Her inner motives would then have seemed in conformity with her outward appearance. But here it was the opposite, and the pronouncement of insanity certainly hinged on just that fact.

Psychiatry was entering a phase roughly equivalent to that introduced to the physical sciences by Johannes Kepler and Galileo. The physical sciences contrasted "secondary" qualities with "primary," those that are perceived with those that lie hidden.

The handful of American asylum physicians that constituted American psychiatry in the Jacksonian era still remained well within the meaningful, purposeful, doxologically-defined world of Rush. For the most part, they still believed that you can tell a book by its cover, a maniac by his anger. Many of them, followers of phrenologists like Franz Joseph Gall and Johann Gasper Spurzheim, felt that one could discover insanity in the contours of a man's features. Asked in court whether he could diagnose insanity just by looking, Amariah Brigham of Utica Asylum pointed out a balcony spectator and pronounced him insane. The luckless man was rushed to the nearest asylum.[17] The new demonology was but one part of the physicians' effort to save their doxologically-defined world.

The physicians reacted to the unpredictable and unaccountable actions of those described as morally insane with the same distress as had Prichard. Such acts seemed to them like explosions coming from the depths of the earth. Isaac Ray spoke of the "act of violence, unprovoked by any adequate cause, and at variance with the [individual's] character and disposition, coming like thunder from a cloudless sky. . . . " John Butler, in a report from his Hartford Retreat, wrote of delusions " 'cropping out,' as the geologists would say, without any indications as to the ordinary formulation of the daily life to lead us to expect it." The *American Journal of Insanity*, under Brigham's editorship, reprinted the words of a French physician to the effect that a "horrible act, a murder, an arson, committed without cause and without motives of interest, by an individual whose actions have been previously correct, must be the result of insanity."[18]

To the physicians of the 1840s and 1850s some hidden agent was at work. But what kind of agent? The physicians struggled. Ray described it as a "feeling contemplated with horror, and successfully resisted, until at last, having steadily increased its strength, it bore down all opposition." Butler imagined a "latent power ... run wild with mischief," and said "this powerful and irresponsible agent should never be ignored." The alien agent was variously described as the "insane diathesis," a "scrofulous taint of the system," an inherited "germ of disease," or simply as the "morbid germ." Ray called it the "intrusion of a foreign element," explaining that this "insane temperament," is "hidden from the senses, and beyond the reach of the scalpel or microscope."[19] Insanity was becoming less and less a condition of the personality and more and more an external force acting upon and controlling it.

The doxologically-defined world stood violated by events that, being unexpected and inexplicable, violated perceptual control. Lawfulness seemed lost unless insanity was recognized as *simply* a physical disease. Purpose and design were lost from the world *if* insanity was recognized as simply a physical disease. But the notion of the irrational as a force offered a way out, a way that would give the irrational a context, a meaning, and a purpose, thus saving the doxological approach. The irrational could be made into a new demonism, part of a new moral allegory, if the disease agent could be opposed by a principle for good with which it is locked in mighty combat. O. W. Morris, of the New York Deaf and Dumb Institution, described a "vital principle" that provides energy to the body and brain, and which, when depleted, opens the way to insanity. Ray argued that the turmoil of modern life eats away at the "vital energies" and that the "atmosphere of excitement" of modern times "is calculated to impair the vigor of the mind and facilitate the invasion of disease." T. R. H. Smith, superintendent at the Jefferson, Missouri, asylum, reported that too much youthful expenditure of the brain's energy enables "disease tendencies [to] gain the ascendency in their struggle with the vital powers, and the equilibrium being disturbed, hereditary diseases begin to claim their victims. . . . " Supporters of the moral insanity doctrine were thus drawn in on the side of vitalism in the contemporary mechanist-vitalist debate. Supporters of vitalism leaned upon materialist doctrine, the belief (drawing on Newton's notion of the aether) in substantial fluid-like forces invisibly at work in the world, while mechanism countered with Newtonian corpuscular theory to explain all motion in terms of primary particles, their com-

bination into masses, and the forces of attraction and repulsion between them.[20]

The next major step in the evolution of the moral insanity idea — a step pregnant with implication for the new demonism — was being prepared in mid-century France in the twin ideas of "degeneracy" and the "savage." Prichard had used those ideas in explaining why certain races or cultures seem more primitive than others, but their application to the idea of insanity awaited the hand of Benedict Morel, whose *Clinical Studies* (1852, 1853) and *Treatise on Physical, Intellectual, and Moral Degeneracy* (1857) argued that the insane share the characteristics of degeneracy with savage races: "Such temperament, such intellectual or moral aptitude, such quality or such physical defect, are the privileges, or, if one wishes, the characteristic elements of certain families and even of certain races."[21] A fateful marriage of ideas, this! A fateful interweaving of two sciences. The new demonism discovered its metaphor, the "savage." Thus reinforced, the concept of moral insanity was to become the vessel in which the doxological approach remained afloat in the hostile waters of the twentieth century. Our attention must now turn to a group of American asylum physicians who armed themselves with a full-fledged mechanistic philosophy and marched against the moral insanity doctrine.

The physicians who dominated the American psychiatric scene to mid-century had been a fairly homogeneous lot, a like-minded group of reformers. They pioneered in the planning and organization of the new asylums. They agreed, generally speaking, on the truth of the moral insanity concept. They supported each other's efforts in the courts. They had developed enough professional identity to organize the Association of Medical Superintendents of American Institutions for the Insane. Their moral-treatment approach to therapy defined their institutions as asylums, not as prisons. Their aim was to blend healing with reform, not incarceration.

But the passing years took their toll. The asylums became overcrowded. The press and public reacted heatedly against the insanity plea. The psychiatrists and their institutions became centers of a political whirlwind. The older men were soon succeeded by superintendents who tended to be administrators and able politicians, skeptical of the doctrine of moral insanity and doubtful of the alleged power of nature to heal. Of all the new physicians, one stands out as representative: John Gray of Utica Asylum, who was to symbolize the reaction against the new doctrine of insanity.[22]

Gray took over the asylum at Utica in 1855, falling heir to the strategically important *American Journal of Insanity* that his predecessor, Amariah Brigham, had established there in 1844. From the outset of his editorship, Gray went head-on against the grand old man of the moral insanity persuasion, Isaac Ray, and in the process arrogated to himself the role of defender of religion, public morals, and the true science. His following within the association grew, and the decades following the Civil War belonged largely to it.

Gray's theoretical position was that insanity is simply and solely a matter of somatic disease. For him this truth had two profound implications: there can be no disease affecting the human soul, and there can be no breaks in the order of nature, no freak, indeterminate happenings. In his eyes, to allow ruptures in the rigid order of nature was atheism. He was a thoroughgoing determinist who wanted people punished for their sins. He also saw the problem in his position. His solution held enormous implications for future American psychiatry.

In 1856 a young lady ("Miss C") came to Gray's asylum for help in controlling her murderous impulses. Some years before she had been compelled to put aside all prospects of marriage so that she might care for and support her parents in their upstate New York home. Before too long she began hearing voices and after the custom of the time became a Spiritualist, edifying her neighbors with local gossip and predictions of the future. But the voices were less concerned with her neighbors than with her own situation. They began to urge violence against her parents. When she refused, they urged self-destruction. Desperately afraid, she put herself under Gray's protection.

Because it was so clearly the sort of case his enemies were using to support their claims, Gray took an immediate interest. He noticed that during her periods of violence Miss C lost consciousness of the fact that the voices were really alien to herself. He noticed also that upon recovery Miss C would once again realize the true nature of the voices. The evidence seemed conclusive to Gray: the emotions and the intellect are functions of the physical brain (to that extent Ray was right), but the human will is *not* a function of the brain, the will has no physical basis whatever; it is the true moral agent. So, though Miss C's intellect and emotions had been victimized by physical disease (Gray inferred its presence), the will yet remained free to exercise its control up to the moment of violence. Miss C was insane only during those moments when the will was itself lost to disease.

Gray felt he had isolated and defined the spiritual element in man — that immaterial part that lies beyond the reach of disease. With her ability to stand outside her delusions during periods of calm, Miss C gave him his key: one can somehow stand outside one's own ideas; there is a self that is separate from and beyond one's ideas and their organic base. So Gray defined the will as this ability to exercise self-control by standing outside oneself in an attitude of self-objectification and self-manipulation. He called his version of the will the "conscious ego." He wrote that though "the noblest results of the reason and imagination must be considered the products of a natural organ, the will, the conscious *ego*, remains independent of the organ, in its existence." Insanity, he concluded, is more than the sort of delusion characteristic of Spiritualism, more than the loss of reason, and more than abnormal passion. Insanity involves the loss of selfhood.[23]

Gray's writings glow with self-satisfaction. He was sure he was saving the spiritual element in man from its detractors. But was he? His conscious ego was not in fact an essential thing like a "soul." It was instead a "self," a thing which comes and goes, and may even (in insanity) flicker out. And his insane person was denuded of that self — that vaunted spiritual element. Gray's insane person was a mere physical object, a thing blindly and randomly obeying the laws that control matter. It was a completely dehumanized vision of man.

The charges Gray and his friends directed against their opponents simply exposed their own confusion. They had painted a reductionist picture of man, but by making it seem a portrait of insanity, they were able to persuade themselves that the reductionist implications of their mechanism do not apply to the sane. Their tactic was to become a hallmark of American psychiatry. By contrasting sanity with the reductionist vision of man, psychiatry came to believe it held in its hands the power to save man's humanity. Armed with their conscious ego idea, psychiatrists would contend that, excepting the insane, mankind has risen above the level of the savage and the machine. And that argument was to be expanded and elaborated endlessly. It would be argued that the spiritual estate of true humanity involves an evolutionary advance out of savagery, and that the nonhuman condition of insanity is a degeneration backward down the ladder of evolution. Before long, Morel's idea of degeneracy would be used in a way that made it indistinguishable from reductionism. Gray's reductionism made the insane person a machine, Morel's made him a savage. The later term "regression" would come to embody both ideas.

Gray's *American Journal of Insanity* kept the profession in constant touch with developments in English reflex-arc physiology—by mid-century well-developed by Charles Bell, Marshall Hall, Thomas Laycock, and Gray's own favorite, William Carpenter[24]—and those social philosophers who were willing to put that physiology to work.[25] Gray believed the work of these men was destined to save his science. But what it really did was to plunge the science of man into the scientific universe defined by Galileo, René Descartes, Isaac Newton, and John Locke, featuring as its point of departure the Cartesian dualism in which each person is tightly locked into the prison of his own private sensations. What Gray could not notice was that he had adopted a philosophy that exactly reflected his own perceptual events. The Cartesian dualism, when rigidly defined by mechanism, relegated that which is directly perceived to the realm of fleeting, ephemeral appearances, just as Miss C's selfhood faded away before his eyes.

Both sides of the controversy over moral insanity made the same basic decision, to look for a reality—be it the demonic or the automaton—behind the patient's surface appearance. Behind the facade of selfhood seemed to lurk a not-self, either some demon of evil or some nonhuman machine—physicians' constructs impregnated with their forebodings in the face of randomness. The new essence that the patient seemed to present was a total lack of essence. The psychiatric consciousness was shifting from Rush's easy person-person relation and trust in one's perceptions, to the doctor-patient relation, in which the scientist intervenes with his arsenal of constructs, his reconstructions, and his objectivity. The not-self, which the physician had discovered in his patient, was actually his own alienation from the patient as a person. His discovery of the not-self was his discovery of and disguise for his own alarm. The project for future psychiatry was thus set: to complete the disowning process; to get the patient to accept the not-self as his own.

In the 1860s the physicians' metaphors for this not-self were still inchoate and tentative, lacking the definition and power they would have when incorporated into an ideology. It is to this important next step that we now turn.

Taken as a cultural ideal, the notion of being "genteel" was the late nineteenth century's attempt to recapture the earlier American concept of the "gentleman." The gentleman had flourished in the upper social reaches of mercantile capitalism as the quintessence of manners and morals. The idea of the natural gentleman had a democratic flavor: one was a gentleman by nature rather than by social position.[26] We note how easily the concept of the natural gentleman fit in with the doxological style. It assumed gentility as an essence.

The gentleman ideal, born and nurtured in the rural community and the town, did not long survive the onslaught of industrialization. Because his position relied on the sort of deference characteristic of tradition-directed controls, the gentleman became a casualty of the trend toward inner-directedness as well as the anti-aristocratic political rhetoric of the Jacksonian era.[27] As industrialization gained momentum following the Civil War, he was displaced from economic and political power. The cultural ideal that defined him had no secure place in the industrial capitalist-proletariat context. There seemed precious little of gentility among the new barons of finance and industry or among the crowds of city workers. For their part, the gentlemen professionals were on the verge of making the transition to roles defined by technical proficiency. But for that period spanning the last three decades of the nineteenth century, the cultural ideal that had defined the gentleman lingered and produced the phenomenon we know as the "genteel."

Historian Stow Persons has described the genteel sense of being afloat in the seas of mass society. Edwin Lawrence Godkin, editor of the *Nation*, began to feel that his period was analogous to the Dark Ages: a civilization beset by barbarians. Henry Adams grew convinced that Americans were losing their individuality in an amorphous mass. Charles Eliot Norton, with his 1853 *Considerations on Some Recent Social Theories*, began his lifelong tendency to divide American society into the classes and the masses, a small civilized minority confronted by a rising tide of barbarism.[28]

Persons agrees that American society was evolving into something we are obliged to call "mass" society. But a look at the metaphors and mythology rising in genteel psychiatry suggests a different interpretation. Unable to find a class definition for themselves within the context of industrial capitalism, the genteel sought alternative contexts, one of which was supplied by psychiatry and reflected a tendency to seek class redefinition in psychological terms by pitting the "sane" genteel against the less-than-sane crowd man.

One of the best windows into the late-nineteenth-century genteel (and neurological) mind is opened for us in the fictional works of neurologist S. Weir Mitchell, the wealthiest and most sought-after physician in all Philadelphia. His fame among his fellow neurologists rested on a number of practical manuals on the treatment of nervousness and his celebrated rest cure. But it was in his fiction that he became something of a schoolmaster to his class.

Mitchell's genteel ladies and gentlemen had a mission: they were to be the country's social conscience. Mitchell helped his class discover that its cultural attainments had given it a higher humanity and a destiny. But just beneath the surface of this smugness lay a gnawing uncertainty.

It was the age of Darwin. The doxological approach was faltering. Instead of a natural and essential gentility, one was faced with the vision of a lurking savage within. As often as he sounded the theme of a genteel mission, Mitchell played on the theme of self-control. When his tragic heroine, Constance Trescot, saw her husband shot down in cold blood, she turned into a monomaniac of revenge. She lost self-control, became driven. Making the murderer Grayhurst her prey, she shadowed him by day, haunted him by night. In his turn, he was pushed to the edge of insanity. For Grayhurst, Mitchell, and the genteel, insanity was a nameless horror. Discovering the shadow of the insane Constance upon him, Grayhurst "longed to look back at her. . . . Now for the first time, he felt fear in its purity. . . . What did he now dread? He did not know. . . . These revelations of what lies hidden in the abysses of the mind are, at times, startling evidence of how little we know of the world of the self."[29]

Insanity brought to mind that dark and windowless thing, the abyss.

John Sherwood, Ironmaster confronts us with "the terrible abyss of an insane mind" as the maniac Hapworth made his solitary flight into the Maine woods night only to plunge headlong into a giant gorge: "He caught that maple sapling as he went over and held on. Then it broke, as you can see, when he swung out over the abyss. . . . By heavens! in the darkness. . . ."[30] The genial Dr. North of another book, and Mitchell's self-portrait, spoke thus: "There are times when I seem to hang awed over the abyss of my own mind, with wonder near akin terror."[31] Mitchell wrote no deathless prose, but he did sufficiently hint of the shadow that was crossing the genteel mind.

Mitchell sensed the isolation that historian Persons found in the socially mobile but nongenteel characters of William Dean Howells' fiction. Mitchell's iron-manufacturing John Sherwood awoke to the fact that human sympathy and companionship were being driven from his life by his labors. Fearing that he was becoming little more than a thinking automaton, Sherwood dropped everything and retired to the woods for self-renewal. Mitchell knew that, if he were pushed further, Sherwood would have become one of the insane, an automaton locked into his own fixed ideas. In Mitchell's work the "abyss" was insanity, the extreme form of isolation, the total contrast to the open and friendly society of the genteel.

There was thus this troubled underside to the genteel mind. The dream-entrapped automatons of Ambrose Bierce and Mark Twain haunted it. While the Horatio Algers and Lyman Abbotts, the Russell Conwells and Henry Ward Beechers talked of Christianizing the marketplace and heralded the family as a haven of mutual sympathy and sensitivity, the age imprisoned its genteel wives and daughters in corsets and lace that their bodies might be hidden from view. Darwin had exposed man's animality. Physicians began to preach the pathological nature of female sexuality. Writers, ranging from Bierce and Twain to Howells and Henry James, began to think of human lovemaking as gross, animal copulation. Further, Darwin brought man into scientific naturalism's vision of a world composed solely of detached and discrete objects, each hanging in dumb isolation in the great void of space. The vision of the nonhuman lurked beneath Alger's optimism and Howells' accent on the "more smiling aspects" of life. It was given to the neurologists to help their age fend it off.

As the genteel began to turn to neurologists for spiritual advice and class definition, they discovered "nervousness." Prostrate ladies and gentlemen began to litter the nineteenth-century stage. Leading figures among the genteel, men such as William James, Horace Bushnell, Charles Eliot Norton, neurologists such as James Jackson Putnam, Morton Prince, and Mitchell himself, found themselves compelled to grope their ways through waves of exhaustion and depression. The New York City neurologist George Beard set things in motion. He had read an obscure 1868 report from Michigan describing the nervousness of isolated farm wives as "neurasthenia." In 1869, ignoring the farm wives, Beard told the readers of the *Boston Medical and Surgical Journal* that he had discovered the malady of the genteel. In his hands nervous prostration became the plight of the most highly civilized; the plight, that is, of those who overwork the higher nervous centers of the brain.

The idea behind neurasthenia was not new. For Ray's "vital powers" Beard substituted "nerve force." For Ray's inner-directed man, exhausting himself with ambition, Beard substituted the extreme refinement of the genteel. While others talked of cerebral exhaustion due to deficient or impure blood supply, Beard spoke of overtaxed nervous energy reserves. But Beard made a vital departure. No longer was it to be a matter of a disease germ stealthily ripening in a few unfortunates; now one was susceptible to degeneration simply by virtue of belonging to a class.[32]

The times were ready for Beard's idea. It drew from both sides of the moral insanity controversy. On one side it pictured the exhausted sufferer as an automaton lacking higher consciousness. On the other, it pictured a savage agent just beneath the surface of consciousness waiting to spring and usurp the throne of reason, once the higher, controlling powers of the mind exhaust themselves.

Moreover, supporting ideas for Beard's notions were coming in profusion from the European continent. I have mentioned Morel's preliminary identification between savagery and insanity as the twin fruits of degeneration. Very quickly a school of thought developed around the idea, centered on the work of Nordau, Krafft-Ebing, and Lombroso. Meanwhile, Jacques-Joseph Moreau (de Tours), working with the hallucinatory substance, hachish, convinced himself of the close correlation between dreaming and insanity. And across the English Channel, the physician John Hughlings Jackson was working out a description of the nervous system to conform with the evolutionary theory being elaborated by his friend Herbert Spencer. Jackson's nervous system was a series of "levels," from lower to higher, each constituting a stage in the integration of sensory input. He described the right hemisphere—a lower level—as the region of dreams. If the rational level situated in the left hemisphere loses its powers, one slips backward on the evolutionary scale to the right hemisphere. In the heat of contemporary speculation, Jackson's lower levels were inevitably equated with the savage mind.[33]

American psychiatry's claims to originality were modest. The moral insanity concept came from England. John Gray's position was foreshadowed by Carpenter's in England, who wrote that "So far as the directing influence of the will over the current of thought is suspended, the individual becomes a thinking automaton. . . . "[34] The higher-lower doctrine got its formal theoretic statement by Hughlings Jackson. But such precedents do not tell the whole story. They were borrowings with which to clothe American perceptions. When, for example, Hughlings Jackson's evolutionary statement got its first airing in America, a writer for the *Journal of Nervous and Mental Disease* insisted that "Stripped of evolutionary verbage the views of Dr. Hughlings Jackson . . . simply amount to the same statement made by hundreds of alienists since the dawn of psychiatry, that delusions, hallucinations, insane conduct, etc., result from inhibitions having been removed by disease. Insanity removes the chains, and the savage in man springs to the surface."[35]

Of course it was not true that alienists since the dawn of psychiatry had been saying just that. Ray had never spoken of a savage, nor had Gray. Nor had their colleagues. They had spoken of hidden forces, however, and of alien agents, reduced consciousness, and the like. They had seeded the ground for the American reception of Hughlings Jackson, and, later, of Freud.

And the neurologists in America reaped the harvest. Lurid descriptions thickened the air from the 1870s onward. The *Boston Medical and Surgical Journal,* for example, in 1881 endorsed as the "most enlightened thought" of the day an editorial from England to the effect that "First in order go the higher moral qualities of the mind, next those which are the result of personally formed habits. . . . At length the polish which civilization gives to humanity is lost . . . until

[man] is reduced to the level of a creature inspired by purely animal passions, and obeying the lower brutish instincts."[36] New York City neurologist Edward Spitzka described an epileptic as looking "like nothing so much as a wild beast driven to the verge of savage ferocity," and in another place mused that the "wild beast . . . is slumbering in us all." Theodore Fisher of Boston described the affects of "anemia" or "plethora" of the blood on the "supreme nervous centres" as causing the individual to "become the slave of impulses the most vile." J. S. Wight, believing that he had found the criminal type, warned that the "last developed sense, the moral sense," disintegrates first, leaving a man "as passionate as wild beasts in the forest, and as restless as the ocean that heaves at every gust of wind." Speaking of President Garfield's presumably insane assassin, Charles Guiteau, one writer ventured, "It was the memory of a savage." H. Tyler, at Blackwell's Island, reported that "the most elaborate and highly developed portions of the nervous system tend to degenerate first . . . we see a gradual loss of all those thoughts, feelings, and emotions which mark a civilized man, and those of the brute appear." "Insanity," wrote Beard, as if to sum it all up, "makes us savages, makes us animals."[37]

It does not make sense to say, as some do, that modern psychiatry began with the belief that the insane are after all only human beings who happen to be sick. On the contrary, modern psychiatry as practiced in America began with a new demonology.

A phenomenon I will call the "self-control trap" was at the forefront of genteel psychiatry. The savage passions were clawing to take command. A feline creature prowled each maidenly breast. Primitive cravings burned deep in each gentlemanly soul. The cry of self-control rent the air. But there was a rub: within the context of the prevailing nerve-force theory, the more effort one put into self-control, the more one's limited store of nervous energy was burned up, and the more vulnerable one became. New York neurologist Smith Baker described a patient at war with his impulse to pilfer: "In many ways he felt himself to be like an armed neutrality between two ferocious and determined antagonists." Baker forecast the man's inevitable "neurasthenic decline," because the more he struggled, the more his resistance sank.[38]

Baker called his case "heterogeneous personality." The emerging idea of multiple personality was infused with this rationale of an energy-draining combat between the lower and higher personalities. Edward Cowles of Boston's McLean Asylum described how neurasthenia can devolve into melancholic insanity. Here was the self-control trap at work again: When in a state of nervous exhaustion "as much or more 'control' is exercised, but it requires more effort and expenditure of nervous energy. . . . " Soon, "there is deeper depression, more intense worry, increasing cerebral exhaustion, and lessening mental control by will and attention."[39]

Here was a fine teaching! Exercise control constantly lest the savage gain the upper hand; but in doing so you are inviting disaster. The genteel felt they were walking a tightrope. In *American Nervousness*, Beard put the matter this way: Compared to the savage, the genteel's emotions are easily excited and need a far more highly developed "controlling and inhibiting" force. The higher the emotional sensibility and increased need for control, the more the energy drain: "the more we feel the more we must restrain our feelings. The expression of emotion and expression of reason [for example, inhibition], when carried to a high degree, as in the most active nations, tends to exhaustion."[40]

We begin to see the subtleties of the new genteel self-definition. The genteel believed they were the most civilized group in history,[41] a belief resting largely on their feeling of heightened sensitivity. But it was just this sensitivity that was at stake in the self-control trap. Their advance beyond other peoples had condemned them.

Condemned them to what? The neurologists were quick to answer. A slip from the tightrope was a plunge out of selfhood. Malfunction of the higher centers meant loss of self or ego. Spitzka located the "higher centres" in the cortical associating tracts which, following the Austrian, Theodor Meynert, he believed unite the brain's functioning areas. "Such cortical areas," he wrote, "and their subsidiary associating tracts, bound into the still higher unity of the entire hemisphere, constitute the substratum of the metaphysician's Ego."[42] Selfhood, the neurologists decreed, lies in the "higher centres." Speaking of the higher activity of consciousness, University of Pennsylvania professor of electrotherapeutics James Hendrie Lloyd, wrote: "It is rather a peculiar potency of the mind, directly manifesting itself in will-power; it is the *ego*, and I have been led to regard it as a condition of brain-activity, with its own proper states. . . . Its action is volitional; all other is reflex or automatic."[43] Exhaustion of those precious "higher centres" was held to reduce man to a machine, a system of reflex arcs.[44]

Their emphasis on selfhood distinguished the Americans from their English colleagues in the development of the higher-lower doctrine. The English physicians, John Charles Bucknill and Daniel Tuke, described the insane individual as "the reasoning automaton of wind and weather," and their colleague Carpenter noted that when the will loses control one becomes a thinking automaton.[45] But Gray transformed that idea into his theory of the loss of the "conscious ego." Hughlings Jackson gave the Americans their neurological model for the higher-lower doctrine yet never identified his highest level with selfhood. The famous Henry Maudsley, widely read among Americans, dismissed the ego as an abstraction.[46]

Perhaps because his class situation was more precarious than that of his English Victorian counterpart, the genteel American concerned himself so with the problem of selfhood. The English imagination populated its asylums with "savages," "brutes," and "automatons," but did not proceed from there to develop its fears into a class concept.

The American imagination began to people the streets of its cities with a class best defined by the word "degenerate" — a vast throng known as the "crowd." Beard warned his genteel friends of the imminent danger of American barbarism. Nathan Allen, a Lowell, Massachusetts, physician, observed that Americans seemed on the way to becoming a race of degenerates. In anguish about "unnatural and lustful monsters, reveling in vice of the lowest order," William Krauss opined that the degenerates were forming a distinct anthropological variety of the species. John Chapin, head of the Philadelphia Hospital for the Insane, boldly estimated that the morally depraved constitute about a third of the population. In 1867 the *Quarterly Journal of Psychological Medicine and Medical Jurisprudence* began a short career by asserting that the extermination of the race was at hand owing to "a restless class of indolent beings, living on the lives of others, and dragging the feebler members of the community down to their own level."[47] Walter Channing envisioned the emergence of a "defective class" created by a wasting away of the vital energies.

Neurologist James Kiernan, writing on "Race and Insanity" in 1886, insisted that the degenerates of Europe were flooding America. Irving Rosse, the professor of nervous diseases at Georgetown University, Washington, D.C., spoke dejectedly of a vast army of Americans whose minds are "trembling in balance between reason and madness."[48]

The higher-lower doctrine thus served the neurologists' fears as much as their class pride. It was a neurological scheme that served ideological purposes. The higher centers described the genteel, the lower, the crowd. But to fully understand the doctrine's ideological portent, we need to understand that it supported two scientific approaches, the doxological and the mechanistic. In the doxological vein, it introduced the savage and the idea of evolution from the lower to the higher, giving the genteel their place and purpose in the world. In its mechanistic form it enabled psychiatry to put the notion of "reductionism" to class uses. The two metaphors ("savage," and "machine") became so interwoven in neuropsychiatric thought that their mutual incongruity went unnoticed. Often they were expressed side-by-side in the same statement. Writing on inebriety, Thomas Lee Wright said on one page, "Will, too, [becomes] inefficient and helpless, because the diseased appetites and impulses of the animal being are stronger than the determinations of rational choice—and they rule the life while reason slumbers." A page or two later he gives us the automaton: "Anaesthesia withdraws the nervous centres from spontaneous activity and compels the mind to assume that inferior plan of exhibition, which is merely imitative, habitual, automatic."[49] Sometimes we find the two side-by-side in the selfsame sentence, as when Thomas Davidson Crothers, a leading expert on inebriety and its relation to crime, wrote, "In these groups, the inebriate is a mere automaton in motion, moving along certain fixed lines of action, or acting in obedience to some unknown forces, which not only develop new thoughts and deeds, but criminal impulses and acts foreign to all past conduct."[50]

To a degree, the doxological approach was saved by the new demonology. But it was a limited triumph. The perception of the other person in terms of his essence or characteristic nature survived in a much weakened state. The perception was now being described in terms of selfhood, and that was becoming a very insubstantial thing. Now selfhood existed by virtue of one's sanity rather than by virtue of birth or of membership in the American agrarian democracy. The vital consideration for us is that by the end of the nineteenth century the link between sanity and perceived selfhood was firm. The fact that for the genteel sanity was becoming a chancy thing registers the degree to which the perception of selfhood had become problematic.

2

IN SEARCH OF THE REAL
MISS BEAUCHAMP

The higher-lower doctrine, largely developed around the idea of neurasthenia, was one important aspect of the developing vision of mental illness. This chapter takes up a second and complementary aspect of the perceptual response to ambiguity, the idea of "multiple personality." I will refer to the higher-lower doctrine as the "vertical" aspect and oppose to it the multiple personality theory as the "horizontal" aspect simply as a shorthand device to contrast the idea of the unconscious as a lower phenomenon with the same idea (usually, the subconscious) as a split-off part of consciousness. Until Sigmund Freud synthesized the two aspects in 1900, the horizontal approach carried with it none of the implications of atavism or savagery that were associated with the vertical.

By 1900 psychiatric nosology was in a shambles with little uniformity of usage between institutions or treatises. In 1886 the Association of Medical Superintendents of American Institutions for the Insane dropped "moral insanity" from its official classification of the psychoses, adding "primary delusional insanity" (otherwise "paranoia") to a list including mania, melancholia, folie circulaire and dementia.[1] Many individuals — particularly the neurologists — held to some form of moral insanity, sometimes naming it *primäre Verrücktheit*,[2] a classification being used in German psychiatry to isolate systematized delusions (for example, of persecution) and imperative conceptions (fixed ideas, *Zwangsvorstellungen*). The distinction between the "primary delusional insanity" of the superintendents and the *primäre Verrücktheit* of the neurologists was nebulous at best. Since those (or that) categories (category) implicated the rational faculties or association of ideas, they did not fit easily into the vertical scheme, which, after all, had been elaborated in conjunction with a neurosis. Major adjustments in the nosology of the psychoses were needed to accommodate the higher-lower mythology.

By the 1880s, when the Americans finally had the higher-lower doctrine, together with its contemporary formulation in Hughlings Jackson's physiological theory well in hand, the French followers and colleagues of Jean Martin Charcot (1825-1893) at the Salpêtrière in Paris began using the same data to develop a theory of split-off ideas. Just as the Americans were concerned with nervous exhaustion and uncontrolled emotional impulses and just as Hughlings Jackson in England was concerned with epileptics and their fits, so the French were interested in hysterics and (hitherto) inexplicable kindred phenomena: anaesthesias, fixed ideas, and impulses of various kinds. Everyone was trying to explain the same basic thing—the apparent loss of control in their otherwise sane patients.

The central idea emerging from the Salpêtrière school (associated, after Charcot, with Jean Janet, Alfred Binet, and Charles Richet, to name the most famous) was that exhaustion or psychic shock either act upon one's associated ideas to split off certain of them, thereby forming subgroups of clustered ideas, or act to narrow the field of consciousness so much that parts break off to become independent subconsciousnesses outside the field of awareness. In certain instances, the split-off ideas, standing initially outside consciousness, could assert themselves and become the sole focus of attention, thus acting as imperative or fixed ideas, impulsions, obsessions, and the like. Alternately, the range of the normal consciousness might become so narrow that the few remaining ideas would themselves act with imperative force. At other times, the split-off ideas might get themselves so organized as to become one or more alternate personalities, each acquiring a selfhood. These alternate personalities were thought to be thieves, stealing their content from the primary or normal consciousness. Binet and Janet, at least (and those were the most influential in America), arrived at the conclusion that alternating personalities are characteristic of *all* hysterias and of such allied illnesses as neurasthenia and psychasthenia. In fact, Binet and Janet went so far as to debate between themselves whether or not alternating personalities were characteristic even of normal people, Binet thinking so, Janet thinking not.[3]

Historians trace some of the preoccupations of the Salpêtrière school to the interest in hypnotism begun by the early animal magnetists Franz Anton Mesmer (1734–1815), the Marquis de Puysegur (1751–1825), and England's James Braid and taken up not only by the master, Charcot, but also by the Nancy school of Ambroise Auguste Liébeault and Hippolyte Bernheim and by the English Society for Psychical Research, founded in 1882 and associated with the names Edmund Gurney and Frederic Myers.[4] But an equally revealing line of enquiry would lead back through the developing interest in the dream as the model for insanity, that is, back to the writings of Jacques-Joseph Moreau and his successors. In insanity, Moreau decided he was in essence dealing with a dream-state and, in pursuit of his insight, experimented with the effects of hashish upon his own consciousness. "In some regards," he wrote after his experiments, "the man in the dream state suffers to the supreme degree all the symptoms of insanity: delirious convictions, incoherence of ideas, false judgments, hallucinations of all the senses, panics, outbursts, irresistible impulses, etc., etc." He developed the notion that in the dream-state the power of self-control is lost along with the power of reflection, hence the fixed ideas, compulsions, and associated phenomena.[5] There remained for the later Salpêtrière group only to equate "dream" with "subconsciousness." Referring to hysterical anaesthesia, Janet called the subconscious a dream that persists outside the personal consciousness: "Every subconscious idea robs the principle personality of sensations and images. . . . A dream, subconsciously persistent, in which a motion of a member is represented, invades [the patient] in some sort and robs the principle of consciousness of the mastery of this member." Mental illness (hysteria, neurasthenia, psychasthenia, and monomania) became, for Janet, the state wherein the personal consciousness gives way to the subconscious for shorter or longer periods. He liked to call this a state of somnambulism, meaning both that the subject was in a waking dream and that he had become an automaton governed by various "automatisms" (compulsions, impulses, tics, fits, and so forth).[6]

In 1892, Walter Channing, superintendent of the Brookline, Massachusetts, asylum, reported a puzzling case that he tentatively called "incipient paranoia," because the woman involved apparently suffered from a "systematized delusion," that is, all the parts of her delusion fit logically together making it impossible for her to detect her error. Her delusion was that Channing controlled her mind and will. As she tried to be the person he wished, she became a detached spectator of her own actions:

> She took her food well . . . walked, drove, played tennis, croquet, games in the parlor, etc. All these things she did cheerfully and conscientiously . . . all the time she seemed very much like a wound-up dummy. . . . She acted very much as if it was not *she, herself,* that was going through the routine, but a secondary self she was putting forward, and intently watching, with the hope that *she, herself,* the true *ego,* might be able to do likewise if the experiment proved successful.[7]

Here was a perception in search of a concept. The idea of "systematized delusion" as opposed to the unsystematized kind was supposed to distinguish between those patients hopelessly trapped in their delusions from those with whom one could still reason and perhaps save. Yet the distinction did not speak to the things Channing actually perceived, things that had to do with the patient becoming an object or automaton ("wound-up dummy") and also a helplessly observing subject watching that object.

A variant of Channing's problem was voiced by William Hammond, the former Civil War surgeon general. Hammond's problem was that of "morbid impulse," the relatively new perception that did not easily fit into the context of traditional medical jurisprudence. A man might know right from wrong (thus be guilty by the reigning M'Naghton rule) but be driven to crime by an impulse beyond control. He was rational, but was he guilty? Add to this the idea of systematized delusion, and things got murky indeed. A systematized delusion, being internally logical and consistent, would seem to be more rational, though more insane, than an unsystematized one. Hammond hoped to straighten it all out: "Thus a person who under the influence of a delusion commits an act of violence against another, or himself, is not the subject of a morbid impulse, for he acts in accordance with his reason, perverted though it may be."[8]

For intellectual as well as for perceptual reasons, then, the new ideas from France were welcome. The "subconscious," or waking dream, could stand for the delusion. While outside of the dominant consciousness and while unsystematized, it could account for the impulses, obsessions, and other automatisms that break into behavior; or, once in command as the dominant (systematized) consciousness, it could account both for the patient's apparent withdrawal from reality (that is, withdrawal from the psychiatrist) and for the psychiatrist's perception of the patient as a dreaming machine.

In America during the late nineteenth century, before there was yet a concept of schizophrenia to handle simultaneously the vertical and horizontal aspects of psychiatry's perceptual response to ambiguity, there was a growing tendency for the perception called "neurasthenia" (and its allies, hysteria, paranoia, moral insanity) to blend with and slide over into the perception of multiple personality. An 1895 article on hysteria by James Hendrie Lloyd, neurologist at the Philadelphia Hospital, shows this process as it was often associated with the difficulty in the current idea of delusion. Lloyd, who we met before as a disseminator of the higher-lower doctrine, wrote that the major precondition for hysteria is lack of strong self-control over the emotions. The patient becomes self-concentrated, shuns the society of others, becomes irritable and "not inclined to make confidences" (that is, to the psychiatrist, one supposes). The conclusion, said Lloyd, is that hysteria is a mental problem, but *not* one of delusion: "No such domination by insane delusion can be demonstrated in hysteria." The patient, self-absorbed and weakened, succumbs not to delusion but to what "can more properly be termed mental images or reveries, rising into consciousness." These reveries, in turn, "may be said to be an alteration in consciousness . . . a sort of double consciousness."[9] Which is to say that in hysteria we are dealing with a dream, and this dream can be described as a second consciousness.

The higher-lower doctrine lent itself to recasting into multiple personality theory by the simple device of conceiving the "higher" and the "lower" as distinct personalities. Neurologist H. M. Bannister's 1880 article on emotional insanity suggests the historical continuity between moral insanity, morbid impulse, the higher-lower doctrine, and the emerging multiple personality theory. He mentioned a case of morbid impulse (which he labeled moral insanity) and urged that the highest and latest developed faculty, the moral faculty, had disintegrated, leaving dreaming, trance, or somnambulism as the remaining lower demands.[10] In a series of articles on inebriety, T. L. Wright made the same point. The higher centers become anaesthetized, leaving the individual both "merely imitative, habitual, automatic" and "in a state very similar to the one occupied in trance, visions and somnambulism." In inebriety, the "body is the same, but the minds are two."[11] I have already cited neurologist Smith Baker's 1893 discussion of a college student's morbid impulse to pilfer, which Baker believed amounted to a second personality, and how he went on to describe a struggle between the higher control and lower impulse that he thought constituted a war between personalities.[12]

On February 27, 1904, Richard Dewey of the Wauwatosa sanatorium in Wisconsin met with a new case: "There was a somnambulistic look and expression in her eyes and her face," so his notes ran, "an inward concentration of thought and dreamy obliviousness of the outside world" (that is, of Dewey?). The patient refused to give him intelligent responses to his questions. On the second day she was in a state of "girlish gaiety," and on the third, "gesticulates in an infantile manner." By March 5 her mental state was "analogous to that of a child." Were Dewey making his report a decade earlier, he would likely have spoken of loss of self-control, even atavism. A decade later he might have spoken in terms of regression. But writing as he was in the period between Beard and Freud, he called it a "secondary state of consciousness."[13] Nor was it an accident that he published his observations in the new *Journal of Abnormal Psychology*. That journal's editor and founder was Morton Prince, most famous of all American multiple personality theorists for his study of one Miss Beauchamp and her many selves.

Morton Prince (1854-1928), son of William Henry Prince, sometime mayor of Boston, and Katherine James Prince, graduated from Harvard Medical School in 1879 to eventually become Boston's most famous neurologist. Because his mother suffered from nerves, he took her to Paris for treatment by Charcot, while he traveled to Nancy to study under Liebault and Bernheim. In 1885 he became neurologist at Boston City Hospital, putting into practice the theories of Janet and Binet. Eventually he became leader of what he liked to call the "Boston School" of psychotherapy, which he believed was in main outline indistinguishable from the French School. Working in loose and changeable association with one another in Boston were some of the leading names in American psychiatry: Isador Coriat, later to switch to Freudianism; Boris Sidis, who went his own idiosyncratic way into historical eclipse; and, more tangentially, James Jackson Putnam, a wavering supporter at best.[14]

THE CASE OF "BCA"

In about 1900 a young lady came to Prince for help. She was shy, nervous, and intensely moralistic. Hypnotism gradually drew forth a new personality: "B" emerged, the opposite in all respects to the first ("A") personality. Prince finally effected a cure by creating "C," a composite of A and B. In her own account of the affair[15] C described herself (as C, that is) as completely open and very emotional, which "emotions are reflected vividly in my face and manner sometimes to the amusement of those with me."[16] Treatment had changed her from being closed and opaque for others to being open and transparent. We now have the clue to Prince's notion of a cure.

As Prince described it, C, the true self, developed a cluster of rebellious ideas and emotions that gradually, when she was in her twenties, collected into the B complex. Rebellion grew through the years of her husband's invalidism and death, but was brushed aside. It was the rebellion of a light-hearted girl against a life of harsh obligation. "B" said of herself, "*I was the rebellion*," and, "I think of the rebellion as myself."[17] Those words came from the girl's lips after hundreds of sessions involving hypnotic trance and suggestion. B was the spirit of rebellion, but rebellion against whom?

Prince's description of C's futile efforts to put down B's rebellion shows the intimate relation between multiple personality theory and the (slightly) older vertical theory of neurasthenia: "It is always the case in so-called neurasthenic states that the power of self-control is weakened, resistance to obsessing thoughts diminishes and the latter tend to take on automaticity and invade and dissociate the personality. . . . In other words every case of real so-called 'neurasthenia' and hysteria is a greater or less alteration of personality."[18] Prince, once a self-admitted disciple of S. Weir Mitchell, made the transition from the vertical to the horizontal believing that the basis for the shift lay in his rejection of somatism (the nervous exhaustion hypothesis) to a mentalistic explanation (split-off ideas) of mental illness.[19] However

that may be, what he continued to *see* was not very different from
what Mitchell saw.

After a prolonged struggle, C gave way to B; duty and conscientious-
ness gave way to a child-like nature, or so reasoned Prince. B's sole
emotions were pleasure and self-exaltation. She had no "tender
emotions," even toward her child.[20] Earlier theorists would have
called it a case of moral insanity.

B soon developed a compulsion to aid a drug addict of her acquaint-
ance (despite the lack of the tender emotion). In some way not
mentioned by Prince, the addict precipitated the shock that sent her
into state A, the serious, moralistic and depressed individual whom
Prince had first met. The compulsion to aid the addict continued even
in the A-state, so that A had the sense of being a *detached* and
helpless observer of herself. "It seems to me now," C later wrote,
" . . . that I, while in this A phase, was in a sort of somnambulistic stage
governed by what I have learned were co-conscious ideas belonging
to B; and that the impulses of the B complex were too strong to be
resisted."[21] The statement was hers, but the words were Prince's.
"Complex" and "co-conscious" were pets of his, but I am particularly
interested in the idea of "somnambulism," suggesting as it does both
the automaton and the dream. We will encounter it again, as we turn
to a more famous case.

THE CASE OF MISS BEAUCHAMP

Morton Prince's study, *The Dissociation of a Personality* (1905)
quickly became an American classic. For seven years Prince labored
to cure a young lady who repeatedly dissolved before his eyes. As he
later said, he made his book an intimate personal narrative to con-
vince the skeptics. What he uniquely achieved was a superb description of his own perceptual processes. My tactic will be to run through
the account twice, first with Prince's eyes, then with my own.

Early in 1898 Miss Christine Beauchamp (fictional name), a graduate
of Radcliffe, came under Prince's care. Her problems were several
physical ailments characteristic of neurasthenia — insomnia, aches and
pains, nervousness. But helping her was not easy. Prince found her to
be too reticent to talk about her problems, so much so that he
decided she had a case of morbidness and "fixed ideas."[22] Prince

soon tried hypnosis. Miss Beauchamp hypnotized (B II, later B Ia) opened right up to him about a sad childhood and a tendency to daydream and to give in to her emotions. Still satisfied that his patient was a neurasthenic, Prince used suggestion to rid her of the aches and pains. That worked only for two- or three-day periods.

Determined to get at the root of the trouble, Prince began putting Miss Beauchamp into deeper and deeper hypnosis. He asks his reader to imagine his surprise when under hypnosis one day in April, 1898, this severely correct lady lied to him outright. First she denied making a previous statement. Then she denied the denial. A second personality was evidently present. Prince became convinced when, not long thereafter, the hypnotized Miss Beauchamp began to speak of herself as "she." Thus did Prince chance upon Sally (or, as he first named her, Chris). He began to realize that when under hypnosis Miss Beauchamp was falling into one or the other of two mental states, each having a separate existence and a different relation to the "primary waking consciousness."[23] So now there were three personalities whom he classified as: B I (the "Saint"), B II (later B Ia), and B III (Sally). Prince was now aware that he had the makings of a celebrated case on his hands.

Sally, who seemed thoroughly contemptuous of her other self, was in every way the opposite of Miss Beauchamp. She was naughty, childishly fun-loving and pranksterish, irresponsible yet impish. Prince found her to be a delightful "child of nature"—with a child's mind absorbed in the details of living—quite unlike B I, who could remember only certain important aspects of her life.[24] However, Sally was not the savage of the higher-lower doctrine, she had no evil in her. Prince liked Sally. It was with a heavy heart that he decided to kill her.

Soon after her discovery, Sally was fighting to lead a life of her own and on her own terms; this was to the absolute consternation of Miss Beauchamp. First Sally broke free from the trance state by opening her eyes. Once free, she began to spend Miss B's money, travel to distant places, and make dreaded dates for Miss B with a previously rejected male admirer. B I and Sally struggled for control of Miss Beauchamp's body, but B I was no match, even after Prince informed her of Sally's existence. Sally controlled her through "impulsions," such as telling outrageous lies to old friends. About such impulsions, Prince explained that the individual is often helplessly aware of their domination and that, "thanks to the work of Janet," we now recognize that they can be the result of fixed ideas or emotions residing in a split-off consciousness. This, he said, was the nature of the impulsions tormenting Miss Beauchamp.[25]

Throughout the first year of the battle, Prince still thought B I to be the "Real" Miss Beauchamp. He did everything he could in her behalf against Sally. In response, Sally began an active campaign against him; for example, by admonishing him in angry letters to stop therapy. "I hate you," went one, "hate you for an utter barbarian—and we are never coming to you again." The tone of those letters was proof they came from Sally. In his turn, Prince hypnotized Sally and commanded that "From this time forth you shall be dead to the world."[26]

Sally could be provoking in other ways. Once when Miss Beauchamp was leaving Prince's office, presumably convinced by his latest theory, she turned, grinned, and said "rubbish."[27]

In June 1899, after more than a year of daily therapeutic sessions, a third personality dramatically appeared. Brought to Miss Beauchamp's apartments by an emergency call, Prince was greeted not by the downcast B I nor yet by the impish Sally but by a mature and apparently complete woman of forceful and independent character. Following the first waves of astonishment and incredulity, doubts about his former assumptions set in: Was Miss Beauchamp, "the saint," not "real"? It was a startling thought, but persuaded by the self-assurance of the new personality (B IV), Prince developed a new theory: B I was a somnambulistic shell of the real thing, B IV. Now it became necessary to kill Sally and B I. If this new theory was valid, he decided, then B I was "nothing but a pathological entity, a somnambulist perhaps" and must be eliminated. Further hypnotic investigation revealed that Miss Beauchamp had endured a profound psychic shock some years before. Prince speculated that at that time she began to assume the new and morbid character, B I. "There was no serious objection, then, to regarding B I as a quasi-disintegrated somnambulistic person," and "...B I had become split off as a quasi-somnambulistic personage."[28] B IV had gone into a dream-state during the psychic shock. B I was the dream. Sally was the driving force, B I simply a sort of puppet reacting—an automaton. Dream-automaton: somnambulism.

Prince was immensely saddened by the need to kill B I, but since

B IV was the "Real" self, the others had to be annihilated.[29] Sally, now in desperation, turned her fury upon B IV. Her usual weapons— hallucinations, aboulia (loss of will power), hysteria, trance-states— only drove B IV to fight back, even to threaten to have herself committed. Sally countered with a series of really horrendous acts. One example gives the flavor: B IV one day felt that her feet had been severed from her legs and set across the room. Only bloody stumps seemed to remain to her. Unnerved, B IV declared a truce and joined Sally in concerted battle against Prince. The doctor quickly realized he had been wrong about B IV.

Under mounting resistance by B IV, Prince resorted again to hypnotism, arriving first at B VI and then at B IVa. While hypnotizing various selves, still in the hope of eliminating B I and Sally, Prince discovered other personalities in bewildering profusion. It is not important to go through it all with Prince, but the final roundup looked something like this: Real B (to appear at the end), B I, B Ia, B Ib, B Ic, B II (so far, all hypnotized states of B I), B III (Sally), B IV (the Woman), and her hypnotized states B IVa, B IVb, B IVc, B IVd, and then B V (of short duration) and B VI (actually B II in a new guise).[30] The battlefield was about to be strewn with corpses.

When B IV came under the control of Sally, it became evident that she too was a pathological entity. She was becoming uncooperative, independent, and self-willed beyond human endurance. Prince tried to use hypnotism to push past B IV, through B IVa, back to the cooperative B II. But B IVa's resistance was little short of incredible. Prince was able to proceed only after finding a "hypnogenetic point" in B IVa's back. It was grueling work, but worth it. If B I and B IV were parts of the real Miss Beauchamp, and if he could get their acquiescent hypnotized selves together into one and then wake that one up, he might arrive back at the original and real self; or so he reasoned. And though it took several more years, that is what he finally accomplished.

Prince gave the second section of his book the title, "The Hunt for the Real Miss Beauchamp." I suggest playing the role of skeptic by adopting the attitude that the various selves of Miss Beauchamp existed only in Prince's mind. A new title might be, "The Struggle for Perceptual Control over Miss Beauchamp."

An extremely reticent young lady came to Prince for help. She was suffering from what her contemporaries called neurasthenia. When

Prince tried to probe her thoughts she resisted. Under hypnosis her resistance lowered. This open and responsive hypnotized state (B II) was to remain his ideal for Miss Beauchamp. Evidently he equated cure with openness and responsiveness. Even before Sally appeared to him, he had decided that Miss Beauchamp's reticence when awake was due to "fixed ideas," that is, that it was pathological. His mental set derived from the work of Janet and Binet. As Miss Beauchamp continued to resist, "Sally" emerged—the very spirit of resistance. He had conceptually isolated the spirit of resistance by giving it a name and by calling it a split-off personality. He had been prepared for this when Miss Beauchamp seemed to lie. It was so unlike her as to be shocking. The unpredictable must be explained, and he took shelter in the idea of the compulsion. The appearance of Sally soon afterward explained both the resistance and the unpredictability. The ambiguity caused by Miss Beauchamp's closedness to him was now for the time clarified. He had put a cause-effect scheme to it. Sally was cause. He soon personified his efforts to open up Miss Beauchamp as a struggle between himself and Sally: "My authority became endangered and I found myself engaged in a battle for control; for Sally, having defeated B IV, turned her guns on me. It was evident that either Sally or I must be master." Sally, the demon, became the cause of Miss Beauchamp's personality disintegration, for then she was able to make use of the weakened personalities for her own end. "Thus time and time again Sally and I had a battle royal in which the stake was the control of B IVa." At the end, with his goal achieved, Prince wrote that the "resurrection" of the Real Miss Beauchamp had come "through the death of Sally."[31]

Sally was resistance personified and cause. She explained everything ambiguous and uncertain in the Prince-Beauchamp universe. All that seemed strange, eerie, odd, and bizarre was laid at Sally's door. Miss Beauchamp was truthful. When she lied it was Sally. Miss Beauchamp was downcast; when she suddenly grinned it was Sally. "One of the most curious of these automatisms was the flashing of Sally's facial expression—revealing her presence and amusement—through Miss Beauchamp's sadness."[32] When the cultured Miss Beauchamp stuttered, it was the first sign of Sally's presence; when she misunderstood Prince's commands, it was Sally forcing her to hallucinate other words; when the thrifty Miss Beauchamp suddenly became impecunious, or forgetful, it was Sally. All these "automatisms," these otherwise inexplicable obsessions, impulses, and lapses, were now clarified. Prince's world was not really losing its structure now that he had found the cause.

The word "control" dots the pages of Prince's book. When he first discovered Sally in the hypnotized Miss Beauchamp, he fought to keep her eyes closed so that "she could be kept under control." After Sally awoke and became a threat, "it was absolutely essential that Sally should be controlled." When B IV began to resist, refusing either to answer questions or to be hypnotized, Prince decided that "she always had to be beaten to a finish before she could be controlled." Of B IVa, he wrote in despair: "She is determined, assertive, and difficult to control."[33] The battles for control were epic, often occuring when Prince was preparing to hypnotize (thus control) one of the "selves."

To give the flavor of what was happening, Prince described one of his battles — the attempt to transform B IV into B II by going through B IVa — in graphic detail. This particular fight started with B IV rushing to the other end of the room in her attempt to escape, all the while averting her eyes to avoid Prince's gaze. When he grabbed at her, she dodged, but fruitlessly. Once transformed into B IVa her powers of resistance multiplied frighteningly. It was with desperation that Prince held on to her, searching for the hypnogenetic point over her spine. They fought, they wrestled, they shouted — all this for a span of two hours — before she finally succumbed to his "subtle power."[34]

What was this all about? My belief is that it was all about perceptual clarity. The control Prince sought was, finally, that of perceptual control. The real self would come for Prince when the perceptual ambiguity was ended, that is, when Miss Beauchamp became open, responsive, self-revealing, and predictable. When Miss Beauchamp first resisted Prince's approaches, she became ambiguous to him. When hypnotized, she opened up. When B I subsequently began manifesting unpredictable behavior (stuttering, lying) the ambiguity intensified. The discovery of Sally immediately followed.

From that point on, whenever Miss Beauchamp began to respond openly and compliantly, Prince felt he had the "Real" self. For instance, after B IV first appeared, he quickly presumed her reality:

"B IV was so natural and simple during the interview . . . that the hypothesis that she was the real and original self gained greatly in favor." She became unreal to Prince as she became resisting and unruly. The turning point for her came after the already mentioned session during which Prince informed her of her reality and of the need to kill Sally. When leaving, Miss Beauchamp had turned and said, "rubbish." That was B IV's downfall. Prince discovered her to be slipping back into "antagonism and independence." Obviously, she could not be "the real and original" Miss Beauchamp. Soon B IV lapsed into unpredictable behavior such as vandalism (that is, the destruction of Sally's autobiography, which Prince had hoped to publish), fits of temper, and lack of self-control—all of which "indicated abnormality" and deepened his realization that B IV was only a "sort of somnambulist" and not the real article.[35]

The next "Real" Miss Beauchamp was B IV hypnotized (B VI). As Prince described her, she had no hostility, no reticence; she was, on the contrary, "friendly and frank . . . docile and obedient." This new real self was so like B I hypnotized (B II) that Prince decided there must be a relation. B IV needed to be pushed through B IVa into B II (B VI) and the result awakened. His new theory seemed confirmed when, during the ensuing struggle to awaken B II-B VI, she begged Prince to "protect and control her." On another occasion Prince knew he had caught a glimpse of the real self when, for a time, Miss Beauchamp became "frank and open . . . natural and simple." After further experiment he caught her again. She appeared to be "natural, simple, amiable," and completely responsive to him.[36]

The objection might be raised that it was unresisting compliance, and not perceptual clarity that Prince was after. My answer is that the two are the same. Repeatedly he linked simplicity with nonresistance as traits of the real Miss Beauchamp. For him responsiveness *was* predictability.

A further consideration: it is actually the case that during protracted periods of ambiguity Prince believed himself to be conversing with people (B I, B IV, and so forth) who were not real. He thought them "somnambulists": dream-automatons—pure subjectivity, pure object. During those periods his perceptual situation was not the classical subject-object relationship (the "natural attitude" of the phenomenologists). These somnambulists were not self-conscious subjects to themselves and at the same time objects to Prince, at least not in the way he perceived them. They were perceived twice over, as destitute of subjectivity (automata) and as total subjectivity (dreams). As he pursued perceptual clarity and found it for the time (in B IV first, then in B VI-B II), he was creating residual categories in B I and B IV, the two somnambulists. His pursuit of structure was generating unstructure—a world somehow to be defined as dream. When he had Miss Beauchamp stereotyped as a moralistic Victorian lady, her false-hoods and indiscretions became "automatisms"—impulses beyond her control, so he thought, but really aspects of her that violated his perceptual control. At that point he reached beyond her phenomenal reality for a hidden interior cause (Sally). He no longer trusted the phenomenal realm—he no longer trusted his senses. When Miss Beauchamp failed to conform to his expectations, she became in his eyes literally unreal—twice, once as B I, then as B IV. His phenome-nal world had lost its structure, and he was discarding it as unreal. But it was not easily discarded; it battled back as Miss Beauchamp's sickness. It battled back as the non-Cartesian perceptual orientation, and I suspect that the essence of the battle was his attempt to regain the subject-object orientation—the natural attitude—through the restructuring of Miss Beauchamp.

I suspect also that Prince's battle to regain the natural attitude, and through it his own sense of selfhood, carried him out of the tradition-supported, immediate person to person relation he first enjoyed with Miss Beauchamp and carried him into the role of doctor. His structur-ing of Miss Beauchamp was a process of objectification. It involved a denial of his own perceptual disorganization by attributing it to Miss Beauchamp as her "dream." His own perceptual ambiguity was thereby objectified as Miss Beauchamp's lack of structure or selfhood. He found his security and his selfhood in his alienation from and objectification of Miss Beauchamp. A structured Miss Beauchamp became so vital to him that he was literally ready to kill for it. The final solution. As Prince described it, a feeling, thinking self had to be killed: "It was the annihilation of the individual."[37]

But we must not be misled by Prince's flair for the dramatic into believing that B I and B IV were fully real people for him. Neither, after all, was the Real Miss Beauchamp. On the contrary, when he spoke to B I or to B IV it was evidently with the feeling that Miss

Beauchamp was lost in a dream and not really *there*. She was not present *for him*. At such times she was not responding to his selfhood. But once he became aware of Sally and convinced himself that the automatisms were being directed against himself by Sally, he began to become real to himself again — real in the sense of being there for the other person. That was why Sally seemed so human and appealing: she rescued him from Miss Beauchamp's impersonality. Sally made him real again. Sally was his assurance that his world was not merely random, that it was responding to him, Morton Prince.

So we can understand why he decided to kill B I and B IV, the somnambulists. Somnambulism was dream-automaton. The automaton was the world going its impersonal (mechanistic) way without in the least responding to him; the dream was his perceptual disorganization objectified. Those two had to be killed if he was to regain a world that responded to *him*. But why kill Sally?

For this reason: Sally was Miss Beauchamp's attempt to be a person. Here we are face-to-face with the situation of the late-nineteenth century genteel. Miss Beauchamp, as a member of her class, was a mix of the tradition-bound and the inner-directed. The genteel proprieties had become her prison. From every direction forces were at work demolishing the life of tradition and the absolutes of the inner-directed. In her own way, Miss Beauchamp had begun to strike out against her bonds. She joined no equal rights movement and made no suffrage speeches. But she did have it in her to take trips to distant cities on her own volition, to spend her money somewhat frivolously, and even (the horror of it!) to make advances to men. Sally therefore had joined the forces that threatened the genteel way. It was Prince's job to cure Miss Beauchamp of these impulsions, but it took him seven years of hard work. In her timid way, Miss Beauchamp was the sister of Emma Goldman.

Reading Prince's classic is a fascinating experience. One is in at the beginning, where two of the genteel — lady and gentleman — met on the person-to-person footing made possible by shared social graces and scrupulously met mutual expectations. One witnesses the gradual deterioration of the situation. Inch by inch, step by step, as he fought to retain perceptual control, Morton Prince became the doctor, and the professional, and Miss Beauchamp became the patient. Seven years pass and on the surface all becomes the same as before.

But Prince has rediscovered himself as a manipulator and controller. And Miss Beauchamp has rediscovered herself in submission. The modern middle class has begun to emerge.

Before leaving Miss Beauchamp, we might note her words on the subject of her illness, as told to Prince after the cure. "It seemed to her," Prince related, that when she was B I she was "distressed and tired," and when B IV, she felt "comparatively well and buoyant." She attributed the difference, he said, to "moods and health."[38]

A quick look at one of Freud's cases will round out the discussion of multiple personality theory. During the period in which Freud was shifting his primary interests from neuro-physiological research to psychotherapy, he came under the influence of the French School. Study under Charcot in Paris in late 1885 and early 1886 influenced his shift, as did the case of Anna O—a case of double personality— brought to his attention in 1882 by his friend Josef Breuer. In their joint *Studies on Hysteria* (1895), Freud wrote: "The pathogenic psychical material appears to be the property of an intelligence which is not necessarily inferior to that of the normal ego. The appearance of a second personality is often presented in a most deceptive manner."[39] Historian Henri Ellenberger concludes that Freud's methods and concepts of psychotherapy at that time were modeled on those of Pierre Janet.[40] The multiple personality approach was very much a part of Freud's mental equipment.

However, even while working with Breuer on their forthcoming book, Freud wrote two papers, "The Neuro-Psychosis of Defense" (1894), and "On the Grounds for Detaching a Particular Syndrome from Neurasthenia under the Description of 'Anxiety Neurosis' " (1895), which reflect a swing away from hysteria and neurasthenia towards compulsive neurosis as an explanatory model. Like Prince, he was experiencing resistance from his patients, and out of his frustration he developed the idea that was to release him from the confines of his predecessors' thought and launch psychoanalytic theory and practice. This was the idea of defense. He decided that the patient's resistance to the psychiatrist is actually the ego's resistance to ideas that the psychiatrist is trying to bring into the open; thus his belief that the ego itself is a defense system against painful stimuli from within. The ego takes on the task of creating ideas and behaviors that disguise painful infantile wishes from itself and others. Conscious thoughts and behaviors become substitutes for still active unconscious ones. Psychotherapy becomes a search for the real self which lies hidden behind the apparent one.

The case I want to comment on was published by Freud in 1909 as "Notes Upon a Case of Obsessional Neurosis."[41] A young man of refinement came to Freud suffering from obsessive fears for the safety of his lady friend and his (dead) father. Side by side with compulsive wishes to see women naked went obsessions about how his actions might harm his father and the aforementioned lady. These things came out in the first analytic hour.

On the second visit, Freud informed his patient about the nature of resistance. The patient then continued with his story, at points his face taking "on a very strange, composite expression. I could only interpret it as one of horror at pleasure of his own of which he himself was unaware." The patient then told Freud of his "idea" that something bad was happening to someone near to him. Freud's note: "He said 'idea'—the stronger and more significant term 'wish', or rather 'fear', having evidently been censored."[42] We begin to see Freud's perceptual strategy: Whatever the patient said or felt was seen as a disguise for its opposite; horror disguises pleasure, fear disguises a wish. This enables the pleasure and the wish to remain "unconscious."

The patient felt such remorse for having been asleep when his father died that he could not work. Freud saw such a discrepancy between affect and ostensible cause that he was led to look for other causes.[43] Prince exhibited the same sort of reaction to Miss Beauchamp when she acted in ways he did not anticipate: her mocking smile, for instance, or her sudden declaration, "rubbish." After Eugen Bleuler's *Dementia Praecox, or, the Group of Schizophrenias* (1911), the alleged disproportion between affect and cause became one of the classic diagnostic signs of schizophrenia. For Freud, in the present case, it was a confirmation of the presence of unconscious motives. He explained this to the patient, who was soon admitting that his personality must be disintegrating. "I replied," wrote Freud, "that I was in complete agreement with this notion of a splitting of his personality. He had only to assimilate this new contrast, between a moral self and an evil one, with the contrast I had already mentioned, between the conscious and the unconscious. The moral self was the conscious, the evil was the unconscious." Freud, we notice, had joined the horizontal multiple personality theory to the vertical higher-lower doctrine. "The unconscious," he continued, "*was* the infantile, it was that part of the self which had become separated off from it in infancy, which had not shared the later stages of its development, and which had in consequence become *repressed*."[44]

Freud explained that one of his theoretical requirements was that "the unconscious must be the precise contrary of the conscious." He began work to disclose the underlying hatred the patient must really feel for his father. Here something of a struggle along the lines of Prince's ensued. The patient "began heaping the grossest and filthiest abuse upon me and my family"—further proof of the patient's resistance to his hidden hatred.

What evidence of hatred was Freud finally able to uncover? Only this: the father had once (and only once) beaten the patient when a child. According to the mother's account, the patient, then age three or four, reacted so violently to the beating that the father never tried it again.[45] Freud heard this news with "great astonishment." The beating and the child's anger were his proof not only of the patient's real feelings toward the father he thought he loved but for the theory of resistance: "But in whatever way this remarkable relation of love and hatred is to be explained, its occurrence is established beyond any possibility of doubt by the observations in the present case; and it is gratifying to find how easily we can now follow the puzzling processes of an obsessional neurosis by bringing them into relation with this one factor."[46]

In summing up the case, Freud reiterated the multiple personality theme. The patient "had, as it were, disintegrated into three personalities." There was an "unconscious personality," and two "preconscious ones between which his consciousness would oscillate." The unconscious, was the patient's repressed early childhood, "which might be described as passionate and evil impulses." It was just the opposite of the kind, cheerful, and sensible normal state. The second preconscious personality "comprised chiefly the reaction-formations against his repressed wishes, and it was easy to foresee that it would have swallowed up the normal personality if the illness had lasted much longer."[47] Which is to say that the patient was on his way to what was soon to be known as schizophrenia.

Now, to Freud the group of reaction-formations (the obsessions) was constituted the same way as a dream: "dream-work" was the way that repressed wishes get disguised during sleep; the "reaction-formations" are the same sort of disguises in the daytime. The second preconscious personality was the dream come to life. So we get this picture: as the patient sat before Freud, the doctor began to perceive him as a waking dream. Not only that, but more: the so-called cheerful and sensible primary personality was also in some sense a mask (both to the patient and to the world) hiding unconscious hatreds. As Freud watched, his phenomenal realm gave way to reveal not the impish Sally but a devilish brew of passion and hate. Sally was to be seen in Miss Beauchamp's mocking smile, but the lurking, indestructible self uncovered by Freud was too hideous to view directly; it was indeed Sally, but turned into Medusa by psychiatry's greatest creative mind.

There is currently some talk to the effect that modern particle physicists are seeing their own faces in their gauges. Prince had no gauges, but otherwise the figure applies. I have no wish to implicate Freud similarly, for this is a study of the Americans. But it will be necessary to show that Freud's work lent itself to the uses of American mental-health liberalism. Freud joined the vertical with the horizontal — that was his triumph. But the Americans were to take his theory further — much further — than he wished. Freud remained a mechanist and determinist, but the Americans would rework his theory into a revamped doxological approach. Freud, after all, invited this misuse. He was as much an advocate of the new demonism as any American. The difference is that Freud, to my knowledge, never adopted the attitude that mechanism describes only the insane and not the sane, and therefore that the insane are not truly human.

The Americans tried to remake Freud in another way. He did not have a Sally, and the Sally figure was destined to haunt American psychiatry. While Prince was working with Miss Beauchamp, mental-health liberalism was being forged by others out of a synthesis between vertical and horizontal theory. A new class ideology was forming around the identification of the "lower" and the "split-off personality" with the isolated and alienated "crowd man," who walked the underside of the genteel mind. Psychiatry borrowed from anthropology and described the crowd man as a savage. But Sally was no savage, and she, or her echo, continued to mock all the theoretical apparatus and self-justification. Her childlike spontaneity and insouciance tugged at the psychiatric imagination. She became something of a block to the dialectic of objectification. Her presence made it seem possible that there is after all something irredeemably human in each individual's infinite complexity.

The genteel gave us Prince's *Dissociation of a Personality* as an expression of its drive to find unity in growing diversity. But the genteel also gave us some of our great appeals for freedom in diversity. Henry Adams's *Mont Saint-Michel and Chartres* (1913) re-called an age when human follies, mischiefs, inconsistencies, and failures were tolerated for the reason that they are evidences of our humanity. It was the twelfth century, the Age of the Virgin, the age of pity, forgiveness, and toleration. Then, in Adams's account, came the schoolman and scientists—the cathedral-building intellect which, in its attempt to bring all the world's loose ends into one structure, discovered, to its horror, that there are *nothing but* loose ends. As the intellect struggles to patch up its world into one Universe, it builds its own prison.

In the second of the genteel's great appeals, *The Varieties of Religious Experience* (1903), William James painted a scandalous picture in which pathology and freedom are somehow two sides of the same coin. By all the canons of science, Sally was a pathological entity; James accepted this as fact, but he also asserted her rights. If we want freedom we must embrace our insanity.

3

A VOICE FROM THE ABYSS: WILLIAM JAMES

William James and Morton Prince shared the same social world; both graduated as physicians from Harvard College. Both were fascinated by the problem of multiple personality and convinced by the Charcot-Binet-Janet solution. Yet James and Prince lived in different worlds. Prince wanted to kill Sally; James wanted to free her.

When James's *Principles of Psychology* was published in 1890, few neurologists listened. Why, then, do we bother with James? We bother because he was genteel, he suffered from neurasthenia and feared for his sanity; through his experiences we become acquainted with the abyss — that dark repository of genteel fears — in a way that we otherwise could not. We bother with him because he stood like a big rock against the gathering current of psychiatric thought. He at least forced the current to part, to eddy about a bit, and even to rechannel itself.

In the next few pages I will relate some of James's weaker moments, as described in his correspondence and diary, not with the intent of altering our picture of him as the strong and human person his contemporaries knew, but in the hope of eventually relating his ideas to his perceptual processes.[1]

The people of James's genteel Boston world, especially the world of his young adulthood at Harvard in the 1860s and 1870s, were either not responding to him or were doing so in ambiguous ways. His fellows seemed cold and remote: "All the men here seem so dry and shopboard like. . . . Give me a human race with some *guts* to them," he wrote, and complained to his wife of the "cool, dry, thin-edged men who now abound."[2] His letters are replete with similar sentiments.

James was often perplexed and confounded by those to whom he had entrusted his self-regard. Just when he expected glad openness, he met with distance and egocentricity. His letters, especially before 1873, reveal a deep but frustrated longing for intimacy. Long passages in his diary despair of finding such a relationship.

James Ward had been a companion of James's youth. Together they had voyaged to Brazil in 1865-1866 with Harvard College naturalist Louis Agassiz. From Berlin in 1868, James wrote plaintively to Ward that "We long for sympathy, for a purely *personal* communication, first with the soul of the world, and then with the soul of our fellows. And happy are they who think, or know, that they have got them! But there are those who must confess with bitter anguish that they are perfectly isolated from the soul of the world, and that the closest human love encloses a potential germ of estrangement or hatred." His letter then praised a poem by C. P. Cranch that spoke of men as being "clad in veils," which all of our "deep communing" fails to remove; we are "columns left alone . . . of a temple once complete." This poetic expression of failed friendship moved him deeply; he was still quoting it in 1893. It was to be a prophetic sentiment, for a bare year after that letter to Ward, James was writing to his brother Henry that "Tom Ward was here a few days ago — unpleasantly egotistical and ostentatious of his eccentricity."[3]

James, kept from the Civil War by his nervous condition, strove to establish a basis of intimacy with that thrice-wounded hero, Oliver Wendell Holmes, Jr. Following the war the two got together for hours to debate metaphysical subjects, but the relationship remained distressingly cerebral and impersonal. In 1867 James left America in deep depression. From his lonely studies in Dresden and a rest cure in Teplitz, he continued to bare his heart in letters to Holmes, hoping for some show of warmth in response. "I have," he wrote to his friend, "grown into the belief that friendship . . . is about the highest joy on earth." He went on to complain of something in Holmes that put him (James) on the defensive, something that threatened his security. It was an open plea, but to no avail. James finally gave up, deciding his old friend was too driven by ambition, too "cold-blooded," too much a man of "conscious egotism and conceit."[4]

Those were years of search, hope, and loss. James's relations with John La Farge, a friend from 1860 when they studied art together under William Hunt Morris, epitomized this cycle. La Farge was one of those with whom James wished to commune through a letter from the Amazon Basin in 1865. But in an 1869 letter to Henry we are told the end of the story: "John La Farge came in a few nights since. My affections gushed forth to meet him, but were soon coagulated by his invincible pretensiousness. . . . I suppose he happened to be in a particularly vicious mood that night."[5]

After repeated lessons of that kind, James tended to withdraw, to become hesitant and tentative in opening himself to others. "There was," wrote John Jay Chapman in retrospect, "in spite of his playfulness, a deep sadness about James. You felt that he just stepped out of this sadness in order to meet you, and was to go back into it the moment you left him."[6] During the post-Civil War years, as his depression deepened, James became aware that ascribing coldness, egotism, and moral insensitivity to others was becoming a habit with him. He began to think of it as his "antinomianism," his need for perfection. "My old trouble," he wrote to himself, "and the root of antinomianism in general seems to be a dissatisfaction with anything less than grace."[7] Antinomianism became a key word for his self-understanding. He equated it with romanticism, a "nerveless sentimentality" that results in making one's feelings seem more real than events in the world.[8]

In May 1868 he found himself floating in a sea of unconsummated emotion. His "Diary Note Book" contains the following observation:

> About "Vorstellungen disproportionate to the object" or in other words ideas disproportionate to any practical application— such for instance are emotions of a loving kind indulged in where one cannot expect to gain exclusive possession of the loved person. . . . When a pretension of this sort subtly is born in the heart, and circumstances snub it, the reaction is painful; is either what is generally called jealousy or s'thing akin to it. It is apt to become excessive and make one recoil from the object altogether. . . . We throw up the good with the bad and renounce all interest in the object, because the good is uncertain.[9]

The exigencies of his social life were promoting an urge to possess and control; yet he recognized this in himself and recoiled from it. The time of his own personal freedom would come when, having won out over his depression, he would opt for a pluralistic world in which every person is taken for whom he or she is, and in which every person has the freedom to be him or herself.

Meanwhile, as he wrote Ward, he was sinking "even deeper into the drifting slough of indifference and disrespect for individual manifestations of life." He wrote to his sister Alice that he had grown into the habit of viewing society in terms of "mutual disgust and mere toleration," and added, "don't think me soured in temper—it evidently is something constitutional in me." He found himself recoiling from others into a profoundly introspective mode—"*Vorstellungen* disproportionate to the object"—and his sense of the flesh and blood reality of other people was slipping away into abstractions, "individual manifestations of life," mere "forms."

> I may not study, make, or enjoy—but I can will. I can find some real life in the mere respect for other forms of life as they pass, even if I can never embrace them as a whole or incorporate them with myself. Nature and life have unfitted me for any affectionate relations with other individuals—it is well to know the limits of one's individual faculties.[10]

I have been concentrating thus far on James's social world, conditioned by the genteel situation of collapsing tradition and shifting power realities. But for James the intellectual milieu also required new adjustments. While his personal relations deteriorated in the 1860s, causing others, in their ambiguity and impersonality, to fade from flesh and blood reality into mere "forms," powerful intellectual forces nudged James toward making the same sort of shift Gray and other medical mechanists were making, away from the experienced phenomenal realm to those atomic and mechanistic events presumed to operate out of sight. Physics and chemistry, as James read them, took for granted the atomicity of reality.[11] In his own sphere—neurology and physiology—the "school of Helmholtz" (Herman Helmholtz, Ernest Brücke, Emil Du Bois-Reymond, Carl Ludwig, Theodor Meynert), which sought to explain human behavior by the laws of physics, dominated in Germany. A corresponding movement, associated with Marshal Hall and Hughlings Jackson, was making inroads into English thought.[12] James had no choice but to immerse himself in the works of those scientists.

In philosophy it was no different. Here the most insistent voices speaking to the medical student included Alexander Bain and Herbert Spencer, who were trying to assimilate the new neurophysiological knowledge into a philosophical perspective. James came to Spencer in his medical school years as to a prophet, for Spencer was trying to bring a bit of warmth to the world of scientific naturalism. He brought very little, as far as James was concerned.

Spencer and Hughlings Jackson were putting Darwin's 1859 *On the Origin of Species* into the service of the higher-lower doctrine. Evolution was to be thought of as going from lower to higher nervous integrations, from dim and inchoate consciousness to the clarity and precision of the modern mind. The idea that the environment selects from chance variations seemed to give the notion support. But for James this avenue into the bright world of order offered by the mechanistic paradigm was fatally closed.

Darwin's legacy was, after all, ambiguous. His thesis of chance variations could be read to argue that the world is meaninglessly random. James came to Darwin via his family friend, the nominalist Chauncey Wright. For Wright the idea of chance variations supported the Humean critique: scientific laws are merely mental constructs. Hume's critique of "causality"—that the senses register antecedent and subsequent events, but we have no right to call those events cause and effect because the senses do not register their necessary connection— convinced Wright. Empirically experienced phenomena have nothing to hold them together—they come randomly and unrelatedly, like cosmic weather.[13]

When, writing from the depths of his depression, James stated that he was overcome by a sort of "philosophic pessimism," he was referring to Wright's logic. Though repulsed by its nihilism, there seemed to James no escape, and worse, no way to cope morally. Each event becomes merely a successor, leading nowhere. There is no reason to will or to act in such a world. Life is robbed of meaning, for there can be no moral ends toward which events (cosmic or human) might be moving. It added up to anything but an orderly, clockwork, Newtonian-Laplacian sort of world. There loomed in James's imagination the Humean world of "representation sprouting upon representation by absolute happening, of everything being only once, of evolution with nothing involved," at which times "I feel as if the breath was leaving my body."[14] The solid world of the senses, already threatened by ambiguous personal relations, melted into mere subjective appearances, signifying nothing.

In his 1890 masterpiece, *The Principles of Psychology*, James called on psychology to accept the mind-matter, subject-object dualism, and the atomicity of matter as well. But he could not keep himself out of his book; his ambivalence on those questions is everywhere. In the *Principles* he gives us a powerful description of the world as humanly experienced—the "stream of consciousness"—and used all the arts of persuasion to bring home certain points: that the only reality we can know is the vibrant, living one of the experienced stream; that intellectual constructs like atoms are judgments not derived from experience; and, finally, that the ultimate test for the validity of any intellectual construct is the stream of immediate experiencing itself. Yet, despite his best arguments and powers of description, he was unable to exorcize from his imagination the desperate vision of atomic randomness: "the infinite chaos of movements . . . that black and jointless continuity of space and moving clouds of swarming atoms which science calls the only real world."[15]

However others may have received atomic theory, for James it came in the context of Wright's nihilism and his own diminishing confidence in the human reality of those around him. If the shift away from the phenomenal realm meant an uncovering of God's wisdom for Gray, it was otherwise for James. For him it correlated with the loss of selfhood; atomic randomness carried a vision of personal extinction. In 1870, during the days of his bleakest despair, he made a diary entry urging himself "to look the universal death in the face without blinking," and wearily added that "though evil slay me, she can't subdue me, or make me worship her. The brute force is all at her command, but the final protest of my soul as she squeezes me out of existence gives me still in a certain sense the superiority."[16]

Atomic randomness and the stream were James's two realities, one death-dealing, one life-giving. He ultimately resisted Wright, but in his day to question the atomic texture of reality was to question science itself. It took him years of speculative wrestling to take that leap of faith toward the experienced world. In the process he worked a revolution in philosophy. His final neutral monism was a resolution of his perceptual problems as much as it was a metaphysical triumph.

One final aspect of James's dissolving realities needs to be addressed.

His subject-object apprehension of the world (the "natural attitude") was becoming unstable. Under his gaze the object world dissolved into either clouds of atoms or subjective appearance. But when he turned his gaze inward, the subjective side became unstable in its turn, passing into pure object. His world was collapsing into the non-Cartesian consciousness. Two of his most famous essays—back-to-back chapters in the *Principles*—tell the story.

In the "Stream of Thought," the solid object world dissolved into a polarity between the clouds of atoms and subjective appearance. In the true Humean tradition, objects became indistinct from one's perception of them. They lost their rigidity, their boundaries, and their identity through time. Experience became a flow in which the same object is never met with twice because in the flow new feelings and added memories constantly alter perspective. The distinction between subjective feeling and object was lost as feeling became as much a quality of the object as its weight and dimensions, yet weight and dimension are reducible to sensation, which, in turn, equates back to feeling. Again, objects cease to be discrete entities, separated from one another by external relations. Gone is the billiard-ball world of the empiricist tradition. Relations become qualities of the objects, indistinct from feelings; or, rather, objects flowed into their relations and through them into the succeeding objects.

The "Stream of Thought" gained its perspective from the idea that the outer world is no more than a cloud of atoms. From that cloud the senses and attention select the unities and configurations that make up one's ordered perceptions. Objects, their qualities, and relations must necessarily be subjective if the cloud of atoms is all there is out there. The stream, as developed in the *Principles*, followed George Berkeley's dictum *esse est percepi*, and has led critics to accuse James of solipsism.[17] James had no stomach for solipsism, but his object world had collapsed on him.

In his succeeding chapter, the "Consciousness of Self," James turned to uncovering that innermost subjective thing, the "self of selves." Here, just as his object world had dissolved into pure subjectivity, so now his subjective world dissolved into its opposite. He worked from the outside in. Beginning with one's possessions (the "material self") and social relations (the "social self"), he worked back through the personality and feelings to get inward to that inner self of selves.

Ostensibly, he was travelling from the realm of objects into the subjective, but he discovered that all aspects of the self were exhausted before he could cross the line into the subjective. The material self was clearly of the realm of objects; the social self was less obviously so, but James resolved it into patterns of objective behavior. Next in line came the "spiritual self" — one's "psychic dispositions" — the conscience, thoughts and feelings, the will, and, in short, much that had already been described as the "stream of consciousness." Within the stream James found an active center, the self of selves. This, he said, is what we feel as our subjectivity; compared with it the other parts of the stream seem "transient, external possessions, of which each in its turn can be disowned, whilst that which disowns them remains." By this time James had relegated all aspects of the experienced self to the external world — all save this one. Then he went to work on it: "the 'Self of selves,' when carefully examined, is found to consist mainly of the collection of these peculiar motions in the head or between the head and throat." Motions of the glottis, fluctuating pressures on the eyeballs, tensions in the brow and eyelids — such is the self of selves![18]

So much for the experienced self; but what of the experiencing self, Gray's "conscious ego," the "I," Kant's "transcendental ego"? Phenomenologists have seen in James's idea of the "passing thought" an analogue of Edmund Husserl's "pure ego," and have called it a "subjective pole."[19] But such is not the case. True, James would not allow the "passing thought" to be considered as object until it had passed and become object to the next passing thought, but neither would he concede it to be subjective. It was neither subject nor object. It was here that he had begun to break free from the subject-object tradition itself. Neither subject nor object, the passing thought precedes both.

Such, then, was the non-Cartesian vision expressed by James in the *Principles* when he attempted to describe the world science divides into subject and object. When he pushed in the direction of the external, objective reality, the experienced world became through and through subjective; but when he went on to describe the phenomena of subjectivity, they turned out on inspection to be material objects. But always, in the background, atomic randomness threatened to absorb everything. Of course, we are already familiar with the non-Cartesian perceptual orientation expressed in the machine-dream metaphors. What was the relevance of those metaphors to James?

Students of James's thought have neglected the medical trends of his time, particularly the neurological-psychiatric ideas that are the subject of this study. He was, after all, a medical-school graduate whose early intellectual development was rooted in neurology and physiology. In addition, he suffered from what were considered the symptoms of mental illness. My object will be to shed light on the relationship between James's early incapacitating depression and his later philosophy. In the process we should also get a better perspective on the medical naturalism against which he was increasingly to react.

What did James mean when he described his severe mental depression of the late 1860s and early 1870s as "nervous weakness," "neurasthenia," "melancholia," or as a state verging on "insanity"? We already know what the neurologists meant: an insufficiency of "nerve force" to sustain the "higher centres," and the threat of losing self-control and sinking backward to the level of automatism and savage dream. Did James, too, mean these things? The higher-lower doctrine was just beginning to find its systematic expression in 1869 when James was still at the low point of his depression. Some minor detective work will show that James meant just what his colleagues meant.

It is certain that at some time James used the higher-lower doctrine in its presumed relation to mental illness. In the *Principles*, he wrote:

> Dr. Hughlings Jackson's explanation of the epileptic seizure is acknowledged to be masterly. It involves principles exactly like those which I am bringing forward here. The "loss of consciousness" in epilepsy is due to the most highly organized brain processes being exhausted and thrown out of gear. The less organized (more instinctive) processes, ordinarily inhibited by the others, are then exalted, so that we get as a mere consequence of relief from the inhibition, the meaningless or maniacal action which so often follows the attack.[20]

In the *Principles* James also used this alarmist passage from T. S. Clouston's *Clinical Lectures on Mental Disease* (1883):

Exhaustion of nervous energy always lessens the inhibitory power. . . . Many persons have so small a stock of reserve brain-power—that most valuable of all brain-qualities—that it is soon used up, and you see at once that they lose their power of self-control very soon. . . . leav[ing] them at the mercy of their morbid impulses without power of resistance. . . . Woe to the man who uses up his surplus stock of brain-inhibition too near the bitter end, or too often![21]

There was a time when James thought himself to be that man. But did James believe in those ideas during his actual depression, two decades before publication of the *Principles?* On this point the evidence is more circumstantial. His diary for January 1, 1870, notes an intention to read Henry Maudsley's *Physiology and Pathology of Mind* (1867), and Spencer's *Principles of Biology* (1863, 1867) within the year.[22] Both were prime sources of the doctrine in the same evolutionary form that Hughlings Jackson was making popular. Maudsley, in particular, worked out the doctrine and its implications in detail. Man, he said, stands at the peak of biological evolution by virtue of his "higher centres," home of creative intelligence, and the "moral or altruistic feeling." The disintegration of those centers brings degeneration, and "in the deterioration or degeneration of mankind, as exhibited in the downward course of insanity proceeding through generations, one of the earliest of evil symptoms is . . . the loss of this virtue—the destruction of the moral or altruistic feeling."[23] Not happy reading for one who was conscious of losing all feeling for others.

On February 1, 1870, James told his diary he had just "about touched bottom." From that day until the end of April he toyed with the idea of suicide. During those months he read Charles Renouvier's discussion of the freedom of the will and the new doctrine of habit presented by Alexander Bain in his *The Senses and the Intellect* (1855, 1868) and later credited his recovery to those men and their ideas. Renouvier, we know, gave James a new argument for using his will, but how was Bain's theory of habit a saving idea? *The Senses and the Intellect* promoted the higher-lower doctrine before it was formalized by the neurologists. The idea of nerve force, Bain wrote in 1855, demands a new concept of mind: no nerve current, no mind—one turns into a somnambulist. But habit is our salvation. Habit ("association by contiguity") empowers one to act efficiently while minimizing "mental exertion and fatigue." James used the idea and made it famous in his chapter on habit in the *Principles*.[24]

James's chapter on habit argues his desire to conserve nervous energy, but other evidence is stronger. "I am," he wrote to Henry, Jr. late in 1869, "very much run down in nervous force and have resolved to read as little as I possibly can this winter, and absolutely not study." He said it again two months later in a letter to Henry Bowditch, and again two years later when he wrote his brother that "I get utterly collapsed and exhausted with the experimental preparations, and the regular tri-weekly recurrence of the feverish sort of erethism in which the lecture or recitation hour leaves me, cannot be good for one whose trouble seems mainly a nervous weakness, and who craves for sedation all the while."[25]

One suspects that James's interest in medicine was at least nurtured by his involvement in his own nervous problems. In 1863, just before entering medical school, he wrote that his special interest might well become insane asylum work, and later, in Europe for rest therapy and study (1867–1868), he made his central concern the study of the nervous system under Du Bois-Reymond at the University of Berlin.[26] There, while learning that nervous energy is like electricity and in limited supply, he suffered a nervous collapse. He suffered another, the famous one described in *The Varieties of Religious Experience*, which he felt brought him to the verge of insanity, as the result of a visit to an insane asylum, probably early in 1870.[27]

In mid-1869, not long before he "about touched bottom" he wrote Henry that though total rest might save him, he was reconciled to relinquishing "external work" and surrendering to the "subjective attitude." He was feeling trapped and helpless. Three years later, again to Henry, he wrote that his prospective job at Harvard would be a "godsend," an "external motive to work, which yet does not strain me—a dealing with men instead of my own mind, and a diversion from the introspective studies which had bred a sort of philosophic hypochondria in me."[28] He thought he might become well if he could break out of his intense self-concern. He was experiencing the trap others were beginning to describe: the more one concerned oneself with one's own sickness, the less one could resist that sickness.

Like the neurologists, James's perception of the mentally ill overflowed from a clinical objectivity into an anxiety-reaction. This is especially evident in his well-known confrontation with an epileptic described years later in the *Varieties*. The shock stayed with him for years. The metaphors he used are arresting: he felt "a horrible fear of my own existence"; the image he had was of a "sculptured Egyptian cat or Peruvian mummy," with moving "black eyes" and "looking absolutely non-human." James experienced the poor fellow as (lifeless) object, but also with the uncanny sense of a hidden subjectivity; and the whole experience was related in metaphors like those generally in use: automaton, or sense of the insane as object; dream, or the sense of a hidden interior life together with the sense of unreality and the uncanny. Also present was the helpless feeling of the self-control trap: "Nothing," he wrote, "that I possess can defend me against that fate, if the hour for it should strike for me as it struck for him."[29]

A diary entry shortly after his experience with the epileptic reinforces the impression that James had encountered the specter of nonexistence: "now I will go a step further [than contemplating suicide] with my will, not only act with it, but believe as well; believe in my individual reality and reactive power.... My belief, to be sure can't be optimistic—but I will posit life (the real and the good) in the self-governing resistance of the ego to the world."[30] His slow upswing in spirit thus began with a proclamation of faith in his own reality. As biographer Ralph Barton Perry observed, this passage expressed commitment to the moral life. But James's moralism was premised on a more radical sense of evil than perhaps even Perry realized. "Not the conception or intellectual perception of evil," he wrote years later, "but the grisly blood-freezing heart-palsying sensation of it close upon one." That quote comes from the *Varieties*, a reflection on his response to the epileptic. James's evil was a *radical evil*, the vision of evil, as he said, that the insane melancholic gets, and it is *real*: "The normal process of life contains moments as bad as any of those which insane melancholy is filled with, moments in which radical evil gets its innings and takes its solid turn. The lunatic's visions of horror are all drawn from the material of daily fact."[31]

James refused to dismiss radical evil as a delusion of the insane mind. He refused to disguise the exposed underside of the genteel mind with metaphors—the "insane," and "savage." He stood in the abyss, unblinkingly.

Radical evil joined the specter of nonexistence with the vision of atomic randomness. "It is impossible," he wrote in *Varieties*, "in the present temper of the scientific imagination, to find in the driftings of the cosmic atoms . . . anything but a kind of aimless weather, doing and undoing, achieving no proper history, and leaving no result."[32] His evil incorporated the black cloud of random atomic events, the universal death, the sense of unstructure—rendering the living world of the senses unreal. His moralism, if that be the word, grew from his fading sense of self and was powered by the urgent need to lock horns with a substantial world that proved its phenomenal reality in its resistance to him, thereby giving back to him his own reality. If he could prove to himself that this world, by its resistance, was not mere appearance, then the other, the atomic randomness, might fade into abstraction.

James wrote that his reaction to the epileptic led him to an "experience of melancholia" and took him to the verge of insanity. "Melancholia" meant something very specific to him. In *Varieties* he described the melancholic's sense of unreality: "The world now looks remote, strange, sinister, uncanny." In the *Principles* he had tied melancholia to the same feeling: "the complaint so often heard from melancholic patients [is] that nothing is believed in them as it used to be, and that all sense of reality is fled from life. They are sheathed in india-rubber, nothing penetrates to the quick or draws blood, as it were."[33]

The melancholic's sense of unreality was his own during those years of depression and later, when he told George Howison that "I am a victim of neurasthenia, and of the sense of hollowness and unreality that goes with it." This was the Humean world of "representation sprouting upon representation," the sense that "human life" is only a "phantasmagoria" that he expressed to Tom Ward in 1868 and again in his diary in April 1873, when he described his decision to teach anatomy instead of psychology. He favored the latter, but anatomy would give him a "stable reality to lean upon" and psychology would likely drag him down into the "dream, conception, 'maza,' the abyss of horrors, [which] would 'spite of everything' grasp my imagination and imperil my reason."[34] Strong words! James was sincere enough in his fear of going insane. He had every reason to believe it, the science of his time told him so.

In March 1873, just a month before the "abyss of horrors" diary entry, Henry James, Sr. found his son in an expansive mood, "restored to sanity," William told him. Asked the cause, William credited his reading of Renouvier and William Wordsworth and, even more, the fact that "he had given up the notion that all mental disorder required to have a physical basis. . . . He saw that the mind did act irrespectively of material coercion, and could be dealt with therefore at first-hand. . . . He has been shaking off his respect for men of science as such."[35] Shaking off the pall of medical naturalism was making him well!

On the strictly philosophical side, as Perry has shown, James's release from his spiritual slump began when he read Renouvier's *Second Essay*. James found two things there: first, Renouvier's argument for the freedom of the will. His diary for April 30, 1871 reports: "I think that yesterday was a crisis in my life. I finished the first part of Renouvier's second *Essais* and see no reason why his definition of free will — 'the sustaining of a thought *because I choose to* when I might have other thoughts, need be the definition of an illusion."[36] The second element, Renouvier's "phenomenalism," goes more directly to the point of Wright's destructive nominalism. According to Wright, we recall, we experience the world as a melange of isolated and substanceless appearances, "mere weather . . . doing and undoing without end."[37] Renouvier's essay taught James that we do indeed experience a substantiality in phenomena, a something beyond the mere appearance of the perceived event. He learned that the event is always experienced within a context in that it points to the possibility of something *more*, a larger whole.[38] This was the saving argument for James. Over the years he developed the theme that bare experience points to something beyond itself, that the *more* is indeed the substance denied by Hume and Wright. The word "more" is not philosophically imposing, but it opened for James a universe of meaning and freedom. In his explanation to Wright, James suggested this use of the idea:

> To dispute whether Hamlet is mad is ludicrous, if we only mean to say that these acts in the play are mad. We know the acts, and to label them mad does not add to our knowledge, unless it enables us to say that their actor would be likely to do

certain other acts not in the play and specified as *characteristic
of madmen.*[39]

The substance of madness lies not in some metaphysical essence but
in the expectations—the "more"—we experience when meeting behavior we call mad. The "will to believe" is usually cited as Renouvier's
decisive contribution to James. But I wish to stress the element of
substantiality James found in possibility, expectation, the "more." It
was this that James needed in his world if he were not merely to feel
free but to feel real, indeed, to feel at all.

In the *Principles*, James tried to picture the sort of nervous system
that might register a "stinging" world.[40] He argued that experiments
in brain localization were proving that Meynert, Hughlings Jackson,
and their respective followers, like David Ferrier and Edward Hitzig,
had attributed too much spontaneity to the cortex and too little to the
lower centers: "Wider and completer observations show us both that
the lower centres are more spontaneous, and that the hemispheres
are more automatic, than the Meynert scheme allows."[41] The "lower,"
at least, ceases to be the automaton.

James then staked out what was to be a minority position (in the
hands of psychiatrist Adolf Meyer, a vital minority) in American
neuropsychiatry: the nervous system acts not as semiindependent
"centres" or even "levels" but as a whole. At the heart of the matter
was the idea, formalized in Hughlings Jackson's theory of levels, that
a sensory "impression" at the periphery of the nervous system (that is,
touch, sight, sound, and so forth) does not attain full "consciousness"
until it reaches some higher level. James argued that consciousness
begins at once, that a sensation at the periphery cannot be distinguished
from a feeling at the center. His argument struck at the core of the
higher-lower doctrine.

Association psychology, dominant in both England and Germany,
assumed that sensations come into the nervous system in discrete
little units—bits of color, pieces of flavor, slices of aroma, and so
forth—and are hustled up a series of levels to higher centers to be
associated together into whole ideas which somehow replicate the
world beyond, if one is sane. James found it a hard theory to swallow.
He turned it around: sensation comes in all at once as a great
confusing unity, and attention selects out those parts that excite its

interest. Ideas (and mind) are neither distinct from, nor higher than, sensory impressions; ideas and feelings and sensations are all of the same stuff.[42]

In James's hands the cortex (the higher) ceased to be the citadel of mind, ideas, or consciousness. Similarly, it was not a controlling and inhibiting center. The mind does not inhibit certain tendencies; other, more powerful, tendencies do. As early as 1880 James wrote "The Feeling of Effort" to smite down Wilhelm Wundt's widely applauded "feeling of innervation." This supposed feeling was credited with registering the mind's power to initiate and inhibit actions. James begged to differ: no such feeling of energy going out to the muscles exists; we feel only sensations coming back from the muscles and other parts. Then, in 1884, came the famous (or infamous) "What is an Emotion?" which still makes strong men weep. It rejected any distinction between the mental and the physical. The feeling of fear is merely the sensation of quickened heartbeats, shallow breathing, trembling lips, weakened limbs, goose flesh, and visceral stirrings.[43] Few in neurophysiology were to understand his meaning—that there is no distinction to be made between consciousness and the organic events of the body, between psyche and soma—because almost all such commentators have worked within the tradition of the higher-lower doctrine, and have decided that in fighting James they are fighting a grossly materialistic reduction of the higher to the lower. James's theory of emotion was the negation of the higher-lower doctrine.

In 1890, with the *Principles,* James took another step by eliminating the distinction between the object and our idea of it. This, in turn, set the stage for his final "neutral monism," the doctrine that there is no distinction between subject and object, except as they emerge in the act of retrospection. He had concluded that the idea is merely the sensation (or, a part selected out of the total flow of sensations), so it is all that we can know of the object—its hardness, color, relation to other objects, and so forth—and thus, for us, *is* the object. It is only through the *act* that the remembered, secondhand qualities of the object (or, the world) direct us to firsthand, immediate, and *stinging* relations with it.[44]

Each step James took, from the days of agony in 1870 to the relative calm of his last years, developed the point that subjective feeling is not the genuine article; each was a step toward putting the "sting" back into the immediately felt thatness of direct experience. In the *Principles,* he wrote that the sole criterion of a thing's reality is its "stinging" relation to the self. In the *Varieties* the "sting" became the "pinch," and this is what it involved: "A conscious field *plus* its object as felt or thought of *plus* an attitude towards the object *plus* the sense of a self to whom the attitude belongs—such a concrete bit of personal experience may be a small bit, but it is a solid bit as long as it lasts; not hollow, not a mere abstract element of experience, such as the 'object' is when taken all alone." Anything less than this "unsharable" bit of experience is an abstraction, a "piece of reality only half made up."45

Many have rightly said that James's depression led him to formulate a philosophy of action, but we must deepen this insight by keeping in mind just what his definition of the act was. Feeling, object, and organism have been separated from each other by retrospective analysis. What analysis has torn asunder, the act joins together: feeling and object become one again and the individual is brought out of the trap of retrospection, the sting is returned to the world, and the sense of unreality dispelled. The higher-lower doctrine is to be seen as an artifact of retrospective analysis, which, when believed, merely reinforces the sickness it is supposed to explain.

James was not happy with the politics, the greed, or the imperialism of his day. But he left those battles for the robust and healthy-minded. *His* battle was with those forces in the universe that, unseeing and unfeeling, would snuff out his being. He was in battle against the universal death, the abyss. His battle was to force the world to become alive again to him, to recognize his being by fighting back. Prince was happy with Miss Beauchamp, a world that submits. Miss Beauchamp would not have made James happy.

Always on the lookout for the "sting," James began to discover a wild world, an unpredictable and undependable world, a world with its own character, its own erratic impulses, a world bordering on insanity. His interest in the insane took on a new aspect. He began to study them for the insight they could give him into *his* kind of world. Perhaps they could see what others cannot; perhaps they are open in a way that others are not.

James was sold on multiple personality (horizontal) theory and its version of the "unconscious" (as split-off ideas). But his freedom from the vertical mythology enabled him to transform horizontal theory and make it the basis for his critique of scientific naturalism. In the *Principles*, James handled the vertical unconscious quite roughly: "There is only one 'phase' in which an idea can be, and that is a fully conscious condition. If not in that condition, then it is not at all."[46] This, because of his identification of the idea with its object (our idea of a tree is the tree; a tree can be forgotten but it cannot be unconscious) and because he rejected any notion of nervous levels (and their associated levels of consciousness). In his later years, James was not one to populate the world with dreaming savages.

So-called "abnormal mental states" were to become James's personal gold mine. He prepared himself for the *Principles* by reading up on numerous alternating personality cases—Felida Z, Mary Reynolds, Louis V—and even personally explored the case of amnesiac Ansel Bourne. He became famous (some think notorious) for his lasting association with the American Society for Psychical Research, for consorting with mediums, and for testing such hallucinatory substances as ether and mescal on himself in his search for expanded consciousness.[47] He was delighted with his Psychical Research colleague Frederick Myers's idea of a subliminal consciousness that extends beyond the boundaries of one's individually conscious world.

The culmination of all these ideas, explorations, and influences came for James when he delivered the Gifford Lectures at Edinburgh for 1901 and 1902. There, and in the ensuing *Varieties*, he tentatively identified the "fringe," "halo," "penumbra," or "more" that surrounds and leads forth from the nucleus of each experience, with the subliminal. There, too, he explored the consequences of making such an identification.

I have been making the point that when the psychiatrists (for example, Ray, Gray, the neurologists, and Prince) looked at the mentally ill, what confronted them was very often their own perceptual ambiguity, to which they reacted by trying imaginatively to restructure the patient. The point is not entirely mine. James said as much in an 1897 lecture on hysteria:

> There is a deep and laudable desire of the intellect to think of the world as existing in a clean and regular shape. The mass of literature . . . from which I have gathered my examples—consisting

as it does almost exclusively of oddities and eccentricities, of grotesqueries and masqueradings, incoherent, fitful, personal — is certainly ill-calculated to bring satisfaction either to the ordinary medical mind or to the ordinary psychological mind. . . . Everything here is so lawless and individualized that it is chaos again; and the dramatic and humoring and humbugging relation of operator to patient in the whole business is profoundly distasteful to the orderly characters who fortunately in every profession most abound. Such persons don't wish a *wild* world; a world where tomfoolery seems as if it were among the elemental and primal forces. . . . So [their] universe of facts starts with the simplest of all divisions; the respectable and academic system, and mere delusions. Thus is the orderliness which is the great desideratum, gained for contemplation.[48]

In this blithe fashion, James put forward his fundamental critique of scientific naturalism. The *Varieties* merely expanded that statement. As long as we let scientific naturalism define our reality, our private experiences have no footing; our most profound religious and mystical experiences become one piece with the hallucinations of the insane. But let us not so lightly dismiss the insane. It is they (or, those we call insane) who have best explored the experiencing of radical evil. Perhaps it is they who can best define what it means to experience the "more."

In the foregoing quote James was suggesting, as I have been, that in their search for order, the scientific naturalists were generating a residual category of chaos, and then arguing for its private and pathological character. James's position was that immediate experiencing is prior to the order-chaos dichotomy; that order and chaos are artifacts of the reflexive consciousness; that they do not exist as such in the "stream." As long as scientists and philosophers insist that the world is made of discrete objects fastened together by relations that are external and extrinsic to the objects, they will be obliged to give arbitrary structure to the world and will be forever faced with the prospect of the structure crumbling in their faces. This ordering of the world underlies the deterministic approach. Once a Hume or a Wright denies the possibility that either necessity or substantiality can be empirically determined, the determinist is faced with the vision of unstructure. It is by denying freedom in the name of determinism that scientific naturalism is able to set its face against the lurking presence of unstructure.

But suppose, said James, that reality is not the sum of objects, extrinsically connected, but a flow from which objects and their relations are but slices or abstractions. Then relations are not the causal and necessary kind discredited by Hume. They are what is felt or experienced as one surge of the stream passes into the next. They can be the feeling of "more," of suspense, or of expectation that lies at the fringe of attention. They can be the possible or the potential. If this be the case, indeterminacy ceases to stand for unstructure and comes to stand for potentiality and freedom. Then, the Humean critique opens the world, frees it, loosens it up.

And what of the "unconscious"? Within the context of scientific naturalism's atomistic world (for example, the world of Freud), it is to be seen either as the explanation of all that is strange, odd, and bizarre—hence proof of an orderly and determined universe—or as the repository of the irrational, of the unstructured, the nemesis of lawfulness and order. James offered an alternative. In the stream the present experiencing is fringed about with a "more," an area just beyond consciousness that is nevertheless vaguely felt. The unconscious becomes that realm of private experiencing that can be felt but not put into words—the ineffable, God.

In his later career, James searched high and low for examples of the odd and the bizarre. It was evidence of the indeterminate universe and ammunition for his argument for freedom. Many were scandalized, as they were meant to be.[49] And, as if to rub salt in their wounds, he urged that we all believe in an "unseen order."[50] The question is, on which unseen order are we to bestow our faith? On the side of the rationalist philosophers, the logicians, the mathematicians, and the scientists, their order—their classes or their laws—often find response from the world. In so far as experience repays their ideas, those ideas must be taken as verified. But once we admit that all experiencing is ultimately private and that the laws of the rationalists and the scientists have never been privately experienced, then we must give equal time to the religious experience.

James opened his Gifford Lectures (*Varieties*) with a short discussion of George Fox, founder of the Quaker religion. "No one," he said, "can pretend for a moment that in point of spiritual capacity,

Fox's mind was unsound. . . . Yet from the point of view of his nervous constitution, Fox was a psychopath or *detraque* of the deepest dye."[51] Without denying the fact of mental illness, James was lobbying for the possibility that God speaks most powerfully to the mentally ill. This is where Hughlings Jackson's arguments made sense to James. In studying epileptic fits, the English physiologist had argued that the weakened state of the higher centers allows explosions, sudden impulses from the direction of the lower centers. James simply shifted the context of explanation from the vertical to the horizontal. The more labile nervous structure of the hysteric may well be more permeable to chance incursions from the subliminal regions just beyond ordinary consciousness. He had never quit believing in science. He felt science was justified in calling fits, trances, hallucinations, and the like symptoms of mental illness. But in some cases they may manifest divine incursions. To accept this conclusion, we must accept an indeterminate world in which chance incursions are possible.

Years before the Gifford Lectures, James had written in the *Principles*, that, while the brain is merely a part of the complex of mechanistic reflex arcs, it is so incredibly complex and labile that in it, chance new connections between arcs must be occurring at every moment. Every moment offers us possibilities for establishing new reflex arcs. Each moment, with each chance connection, is a moment of freedom, a moment when choice between the old way and a new and untried way is before us. With chance there is freedom. But we lose this freedom by believing that such chance connections—connections that tempt us toward actions which seem foreign to our nature—are pathological impulses that only the sick act on.

During the years James incubated these ideas, in Germany Emil Kraepelin (1856-1926) was defining the category "dementia praecox" (later schizophrenia) as a steady and inevitable deterioration into madness; others, already discussed, saw in these same people a moral weakness, a lack of self-control, even a regression back into savagery; and at the start of the twentieth century the idea of mental illness as a "retreat from reality" would be advanced by the Swiss-Americans August Hoch and Adolf Meyer. On all sides, mental illness was perceived in the most pejorative light. In 1902 James offered a paradigm of mental illness as a process of renewal. The "sick soul" was one whose deeper sensitivity and insight into reality caused him

to recoil, and carried him to the point where his world literally disintegrated, where reality dissolved. But the sick soul was one whose
"regression" (to borrow from Freud) was a journey towards openness,
towards the subliminal, until such time as he might reemerge as the
"twice born," healed from the point of view of medicine, saved from
the point of view of religion, but in any case, with an expanded
consciousness, a heightened freedom, and a stinging relation with the
world. James had traveled a similar road himself.

James's critique of determinism and his concept of the stream
brings us once more to the perceptual dialectic. The idea of the
stream suggests that our reality is characterized neither by order nor
by chaos. It suggests that order and chaos are abstractions. It suggests
that perceived unstructure follows upon and is secondary to the
breakdown of perceived structure. The perceptual dialectic would
then be said to generate the perception of unstructure by the very fact
of the search for structure. The overlapping and infinitely varied world
keeps intruding upon consciousness with events that do not fit; the
more we press forward towards structure by relegating the noncon-
forming events to residual status, the more we will be confronted with
such events until the residue overwhelms the structure, and our world
falls into chaos. Thus, what was seen by the participants of this
process as a self-control trap was actually the dialectic at work.

But James's career suggests a complicating factor within the dialectic
of objectification. At one point he found himself plunged into a structure-
less world—a world of random happenings, a world of mere cosmic
weather—the world that others, in their pursuit of the dialectic,
objectified as the patient's dream. James opted out of the dialectic,
but not before he brought clearly to view the dialectic of *self*-
objectification in his chapter, "The Consciousness of Self." In our
uncertainty about how to react towards one who has become ambiguous, we grow self-conscious, and our behavior patterns become
tentative. The sense of oneself loses its sharp outline and begins to
blur and to fade. We become self-analytical and self-objectifying.
These things characterized James, and his chapter on the consciousness
of self shows the extreme in self-objectification. There, his innermost
selfhood turned object before his gaze and took its place with all the
other objects in an alien material world.

James's analysis of the self as an object destitute of subjectivity became an inspiration and model for American behaviorist psychology. But the dialectic of self-objectification made its way into formal theory in other ways. It started into operation when one's selfhood became ambiguous. It was an attempt to gain perceptual control over oneself, and the project to gain perceptual control generated perceptual ambiguity here, too, in the area of one's selfhood. Thus, we understand the fading selfhood that plagued James's early manhood. In others, this fading selfhood led to the project to regain perceptual control over oneself by reestablishing it over others. This was the case with Prince. This was the case with the urge to dominance that became reified in the doctor-patient relationship. But there was an equal possibility of the opposite temptation, the temptation towards submission, the temptation to let some higher authority define and limit one's ambiguous selfhood. Thus there emerged the "Real" Miss Beauchamp. Thus emerged G. Stanley Hall's ideal community and full-fledged mental health liberalism.

4

COMMUNITY: APOTHEOSIS
OF THE REAL
MISS BEAUCHAMP

Granville Stanley Hall (1844-1924) is vital to my story. The fact
is somewhat embarrassing because, although he did some work
on frogs' legs at one time, he was not a neurologist, nor was he a
psychiatrist of any sort. He was a psychologist and an educational
administrator who dabbled. Partly because of his dabbling, it fell to
his lot to point the way to saving the higher-lower doctrine for the
doxological approach to science at a time when that approach had to
be disguised to remain intellectually acceptable. By giving the higher-
lower doctrine its modern social statement, he paved the way for the
American reception of Freudianism and became our first high priest
of mental health liberalism.

If monistic philosophy was to be made hospitable to the higher-
lower doctrine, it had to be steered away from James. Hall was the
prime mover. But he never really grasped what James was up to, so
Hall was always at a loss as to what he, himself was really doing. He
mistook James's position to be either a dualism or a Berkeleyian
idealism—he was never quite sure which—and he either did not
understand or did not sympathize with James's rejection of atomistic
(billiard-ball mechanism).

Hall's was the rare good fortune to study under James through two
years of the latter's greatest intellectual ferment. But Hall remained
ignorant of his luck. In 1876 he went to Harvard College as a way
station between a teaching career at Antioch College and his anticipated pilgrimage to Germany and study under Wilhelm Wundt. James
could have been little more to him than a provincial educator and a

rustic philosopher. For Hall, Harvard served a practical purpose. Here he earned the first American Ph.D. in psychology, in preparation for Germany and Wundt. But Hall could be agreeable for a season (in 1880, James glowingly referred to him as a *"herrlicher Mensch"*[1]), and James needed a sounding board. So, for two or three years the two felt a common bond; then the sort of estrangement that marked the lives of both set in.

Hall, who already considered himself an intellectual cut or two above James, established philosophical independence with his Ph.D. dissertation, "The Muscular Perception of Space," partially published in 1878. His statement that "Psychology is no longer content to hold belief in an external world as a mere act of faith or opinion. She postulates an ultimate Monism," shows the Jamesian influence. Both men agreed that the Cartesian dualism is artificial, and James came in for a severe public scolding from Hall when the *Principles*, with its formal acquiescence in dualism, was published in 1890.

Both were after a feeling for the reality of the world—thus their rejection of the subject-object dualism—but each was after his own peculiar sense of that reality. James wanted to regain the "sting"; Hall made it clear in his rebuke of the *Principles* that he was looking for order. When James reserved a place for choice by introducing the notion of chance, Hall took it to be a plea that the soul can interfere in the chain of physical causation, and that, said Hall, "is to invoke the chaos and old night of spiritualism" and, moreover, "ascribing a causative agency to conscious states in a way to interfere with the conservation of energy and belief in the perfect law and order in the brain . . . is, we believe, bad science, bad philosophy, and bad religion." Hall did not want a wild world, not even in the name of freedom. He concluded that his old professor was not a real scientist, because "men of real research work, with a spirit of reverence, and a sense of unity and law at the root of things and pervading every action and corner of space, that is religious to the core."[2] Law and order were Hall's religions.

"The Muscular Perception of Space," which forgot to mention James, was thoroughly Jamesian in its identification of "mind" with the activity of the whole body. But—incredibly—it was also strongly influenced by Hughlings Jackson, whom it did cite. It embodied the higher-lower doctrine in its association of unconscious processes with "lower centres." How does one get from James to Hughlings Jackson? Through Helmholtz, Hall thought, and the notion that the outer world's structure is not perceived until it is acted upon. Hall asked us to believe that individual sensations coming from the outer world remain unperceived and unconscious until action organizes them into structure. He equated consciousness with structure, unconsciousness with unstructure.[3] He had listened to Hume's critique of causality only half way: the sensory side of experience registers the world's chaos of sensations, the motor side discovers the hidden order. It was an impossible half and half world Hall described.

Hall's was a conception of science as an active, aggressive force; an act of the will, an act of control. Not that science shapes the world to human specifications (that, at least, would have been consistent), but that it reveals order behind the veil of unstructure. And then there was James, shoving example after example of the bizarre, the odd, the strange, the unstructured, in his face and asking him to revel in what he was pleased to call "freedom." It was too much for Hall. The science of psychology, he wrote, "is the method of self-control," whereas James's method "is worse than waste, it is philosophic and scientific precocity and lack of self-control."[4] Hall was coming to science for the same sort of relief one might expect to find in wearing a straightjacket.

Hall inhabited two worlds: the chaos of the senses and the order offered by scientific naturalism. He was the prisoner of a mapping which opposed absolute order and absolute chaos, and, because of that, of the self-control trap—the struggle for perceptual clarity that only increased the threat of ambiguity. During the years James was working his painful way out of the self-control trap by creating an alternative to the higher-lower doctrine, Hall was pondering a solution that raised the higher-lower doctrine from a neurophysiological to a social and religious system. To understand what Hall was up to, something needs to be said about his life.

Hall had the gift of putting thirty pages of subject matter into two thick volumes. Most of it was rhetoric. He had come to believe that his rhetoric was the sexual drive creatively spilling over into the poetic imagination. Austere and aloof in his maturity, his youth, as he recalled, was marked by isolation and joylessness. His father was withdrawn, a puritanical farmer practicing his craft in and around Ashfield, Massachusetts. Family social life centered on the Congregational church. His mother was gentle, but not particularly devoted to Stanley. He tells us in his *Confessions* that he became a bully.[5] His biographer, Dorothy Ross, believes that his near manic-depressive cycles in adult years grew from youthful inferiority feelings and guilt over masturbation.[6] His tendency to bully lasted; so did his isolation. His rise to prominence at Johns Hopkins in the 1880s owed much to his skillful machinations against colleagues. His domineering behavior as president of Clark University led to the mass resignation of the faculty in 1892 and to his feelings of mortification and humiliation "beyond the power of words to describe."[7] The catalogue of his professional struggles—the conflicts at the faculty level, the attempts to control the output of professional journals in several fields, even his assertions of priority in the founding of various scientific movements— argue for an overweening urge to dominate.[8]

Domination was an important theme of his fantasy life. It surfaces in some fiction written while at Antioch. "A Leap Year's Romance," for example, describes an on-and-off courtship between a professor and a strong-willed young lady with career aspirations. The lady founded and administered a school for girls, only to find that her beloved professor was having none of it. She was given a choice, either submit totally or lose him. As Moors, the professor, put it: "I am one of those who believes that the highest and most perfect form of emotion is a sense of complete dependence and unreserved self-surrender."[9] The story ends when the lady discovers this truth and surrenders.

Moors's dominance-submission theme became a constant in Hall's scholarly works. He liked, for instance, to emphasize the will, but he believed that the will is best developed by teaching submission. In an 1882 article, "The Education of the Will," he said that a child's "will-culture" is measured by his sense of reverence towards parents and teachers; we "must now compel what he will later wish to compel himself to do." And, he added, for "most of us the best education is that which makes us the best and most obedient servants."

In the same article Hall made a statement that goes to the root of the man. "Thrice happy is he," he said, "who is so wisely trained that he comes to believe he believes what his soul deeply does believe, to say what he feels and feel what he really does feel."[10] How does one *not* believe that he believes what he really does believe? Are we entangled in one of Hall's rhetorical flourishes? How does one *not* feel what he really does feel? Rhetorical flourish or the words of a man insecure in his selfhood? Both, I believe. Hall was not a thrice happy man. He longed for the security of spontaneous and certain feeling and knowing, as did many others among the genteel. So, for direct thoughts and feelings, he substituted the rhetorical flourish, far less dangerous in meeting an ambiguous world that might not respond. And, in the end, rhetoric became his attempt at thought and feeling.

Hall was the product of a time and place in which rhetoric was lush. The home atmosphere was redolent with moralistic homily. School was more of the same. A seventh- or eighth-grade composition of one line shows how he felt: "There is one thing in the world that even with all my understanding [I] can't understand and that is why I have to write so many compositions."[11] Nevertheless, Hall's competence in the rhetorical flourish grew each passing year—witness the following to his father: "I know of no richer enjoyment on some warm summer night [than to] look back on a day well spent, one which has witnessed substantial progress in physical, intellectual and spiritual strength and culture."[12] Rhetoric masked and promoted impersonality. A letter to his sister the same year (1864) shows a consciousness of false sentiment. His and his schoolmates' attempts to fight a forest fire led to this parody on style: "Music of the most primitive kind 'Breathed . . . and inspired deeds of belligerent courage' amid the cheers of the natives . . . while Cilene, the lunar orb, just begins to rise, ardent like a fried lobster." Then he added: "I have waxed thus eloquent in my description to give you a sample of the style of composition we use at this institution."[13]

This institution was Williams College, thirty miles from home. He knew that his expressions of feeling were becoming false. In one letter home he broke off a rhapsody about life to say that "These ideas have sounded to me real and true for a long time but as I read them over they lose something of their force on paper." Another fulsome letter ended: "I hope this letter will not be so inane that it will vanish into thin air like a bubble before it reaches you." In questioning rhetoric he revealed growing doubt about the reliability of his own feelings. A long diatribe to his mother against a schoolmate ended with this: "But I don't know why I scribble this down here—shall perhaps feel different tomorrow." There was also the self-consciousness: "I am almost surprised," he wrote his mother at another time, "that my pen has disfigured a whole sheet in saying what I might say in a page."[14]

Given his home life, it is not surprising that Hall turned to religion in college. One might hope that his feelings in this area were deep and true. In 1869 he wrote his mother that "My experience as a christian has deepened and enriched and I understand more fully the duties and demands of the calling I have chosen." But he ended with this: "But this doesn't sound well-written."[15] He was aware of the falseness and conventionality of his deepest feelings, and I suspect this informed the 1882 remark that "thrice happy" is he who feels what he "really does feel."

We are reminded of James's "subjective carrion," the false or secondhand emotions. Hall's classic, *Adolescence, Its Psychology* (1905), which biographer Ross urges as highly autobiographical, presents adolescence as a crisis of emotion and the turning point from which one heads either into maturity or sinks into mental illness. Two characteristics mark Hall's description of the adolescent mind: first, he used all the metaphors—somnambulism, dream, savage, and so forth—second, it equated the subjective carrion with James's stream of consciousness.

Let me speak first to the second point, because Hall confused the stream with illness. If one puts the stream into the context of the non-Cartesian dualism, it turns the world into pure subjectivity—solipsism. This was how Hall read the *Principles*. The solipsism he thought he saw there, when put into the context of Hall's own system, becomes the input side of the nervous system detached from the motor side. Thus defined, the person is isolated from external order, subject to the chaos of incoming sensations—unstructure. Remember that Hall had split the world into two: the world of structure and that of unstructure. For him, James's stream accepted the side of unstructure as the whole of reality. He had James in mind when he wrote that "dissolving the objective world has become an academic cult that plays on the dreameries of adolescence and robs it of zest, vigor, and faith." He called James "the most brilliant literateur and stylest in philosophy since Schopenhauer, unless it be Nietzsche, whose diathesis his so resembles."[16] James, he thought, was sick, and his psychology the language of adolescent escapism, a mentality from which the strong emerge into the real world of form (read "structure").

To explain the adolescent mind, Hall turned to the current psychiatric doctrines, both the vertical and the horizontal. He had always considered the individual ego a weak thing, forever hovering on the edge of disintegration. An undated speech in his papers pointed out that the "elements of human selfhood are very loosely wrought together and easily break up as in the phenomena of dual or multiple personality."[17] Hall's adolescent was especially so marked:

> Assuming that our personality is compound and made up of many elements . . . into which disease, traumata, hypnotism, etc., may partially resolve it, as seen in the phenomena of multiplex personality, we must regard the adolescent stage as especially characterized by either a loosening of the bonds between the manifold factors of our ego . . . or else by a sudden and independent growth of single elements which leaves their former associative bonds relatively weakened, and perhaps by both together.[18]

Hall repeatedly urged that the adolescent, in his reveries, is a somnambulist. "Inner absorption and reverie," he said, "is one marked characteristic of this age . . . the day-dreamer goes about dazed like a somnambulist."[19]

With one foot firmly in the horizontal tradition, Hall planted the other in the vertical. In a sense, therefore, *Adolescence* was America's *Interpretation of Dreams*, the first full-scale synthesis of the vertical and horizontal. To Hall, Hughlings Jackson was a genius, and the level theory, fact. Hall tried to show that brain anatomy work done by Paul Flechsig, Oskar Vulpius, and Theodor Kaes not only supported the Jacksonian level theory, but proved that the highest level— reason's centre—is first developed during adolescence. But danger lurks just here, Hall warned; the same development that makes reason possible also marks the dawn of "silent reverie."[20] In Hall's hands, the highest Jacksonian level became a two-way street, leading either outward towards (zestful and vigorous) contact with the world or (silently) inward into dream and solipsistic (Jamesian) philosophizing.

Hall associated consciousness with the highest level but never in a way to pin down the word's meaning or to show how it gets lodged there. He used the word in two ways: first, to mean contact with reality; second, to mean subjectivity. In the first and good sense, he associated it with the motor side of the nervous system; in its bad sense, he meant the inchoate inflow of sensations on the sensory side. In its good meaning, consciousness was the way to health, maturity, control: "To acquire the power of doing all with consciousness and volition mentalizes the body, gives control over the higher brain cells, and develops them by rescuing activities from the dominance of the lower centers."[21] We begin to appreciate the uses of the rhetorical whopper.

The model for the bad consciousness was James's stream, which Hall illustrated with the metaphors of mental illness. The bad consciousness was the fall of man from the Garden of Eden (that is, from childhood and the primitive). At this point I must pause to note two things that Hall did for American psychiatry: he associated "nerve-force" with sex, and he shifted the focus of the higher-lower doctrine from a description of the individual nervous system to a theory of ontogenesis, which identified the higher with community (the "great world of soul"). When the higher, with its connotations of selfhood, was identified with community, multiple personality theory assumed a new role. Adolescent self-consciousness became a splitting off of the individual consciousness from community consciousness, just as B I and B IV were split-off from the Real Miss B. "This self-consciousness," he wrote, " . . . blinds us from seeing the larger rest of our selves." And he wrote, "The [self-] conscious adult person is not a monad reflecting the universe, but a fragment broken off and detached from the great world of soul."[22] Hall's submissive urge is evident. One must lose the individual self to gain the higher self of community. Individualism becomes sickness, the lower of the higher-lower doctrine. The adolescent, fallen from the garden of childhood, who fails to make the transition into the higher selfhood of community, is a split-off self, a somnambulist.

Also a savage. Hall did not neglect anthropology. Historian R. Jackson Wilson has sketched Hall's benign attitude toward ancient man.[23] Ancient man becomes the pre-self-conscious childhood of the race. Hall spoke of "unspoiled savages," and the "fact that modern anthropology finds most savages amiable, kindly and virtuous" and "they are only children and adolescents of mature years."[24] When savagery and childhood become the same, so do anthropology and genetic psychology. Wise in one, Hall became wise in the other.

In *Adolescence*, genetic psychology became doxological science, narrative drama, and religious allegory. It described the travail of man—the childhood, the fall into individualism, and the redemption through submission into community. But redemption for the individual or for society was not preordained. "The Fall of Atlanta" paints for us the decline of present-day civilization into decadent savagery. There is too much democracy, too much individualism. Our nation is refusing to submit to the universal "Mansoul."[25] Adolescence, whether of the individual or of the civilization, is a crossroads leading either to community or to a new barbarism. So Hall had a second view of the savage: the embodiment of criminality, the dream, egotism, and even dementia praecox. This second sort of savage (physiologically, a boy of ten) lacks instinctual control: "This man, adult in years and stature, is constantly prone to drop to this lower level."[26]

Sex was the instinct on Hall's mind. Uncontrolled, its titanic force can drive one into criminality. But often it is dissipated through masturbation or promiscuity, leaving one in an enervated, neurasthenic condition. On the other hand, it is the force that lifts one out of individualism into community.

Masturbation was the great evil. It dissipates energy, turning one into a morass of egotistical subjectivity lost in "lascivious fancy." Indifferent to the world, his self-control emasculated, the masturbator's "growth, especially in the moral and intellectual regions, is dwarfed and stunted." Then "barbaric and animal traits and instincts jostle and mix with each other in leaderless mobs of impressions."[27] The masturbator will become part savage and part radical empiricist.

The old "nerve force" was out, sexual energy was in: "Genesic excess, venery, and salacity arrest the higher development, forever exclude the soul from the higher kingdom of man and compel it to dwell in the lower regions, where adolescence merges with senescence." Substituting sexual energy for nerve force shifted the focus from physiology to community. The sexual act became a religious sacrament: "It is the supreme hedonistic narcosis, a holy intoxication, the chief ecstasy, because the most intense of experiences. . . . It is this experience more than any other that opens to man the ideal world. Now the race is incarnated in the individual and remembers its lost paradise."[28]

Such was Hall's solution to the self-control trap. Rather than struggling for self-control and losing energy in the struggle (an individual
battle), one submits to community. "The ontological passion," as he
put it, "culminates thus in a mystic devotion to the absolute in which
the self is forever merged and swallowed up. . . . Further . . . organized
truth, whether in science or philosophy, finds ultimate criterion
in . . . conviction. This at bottom is esthetic, because a logical or
scientific order pleases the mind best."[29]

We are to submit and be swallowed up in order. In submitting we
lose our individualistic, capricious, uncontrollable selfhood. This is
religion. This is science. Impulses—James's chance happenings—
have no place here. The Resurrection (of Jesus), he wrote, ended the
idea that the world is the "sport of malign chance," the notion that
God would play tricks on His Son. This assurance becomes "the
cardinal psychic fact of early Christiandom."[30] In their mutual elimination of chance, science and Christianity become one:

> Science . . . is the most precious achievement of the race thus
> far. It has made nature speak to man with the voice of God, has
> given man prevision so that he knows what to expect in the
> world, has eliminated shock, and, above all, has made the world
> a uni-verse coherent and consistent throughout . . . a great whole
> with a logical character, working in every part, could we but
> know it, with the exactness and regularity of a machine.[31]

Hall's community, his "higher," was not essentially different from
those proposed by other intellectuals of the progressive era: Josiah
Royce, John Dewey, George Herbert Mead. Like Hall, these men
started their careers from a German idealist base. Rail against absolutes though they might, they labored to make new ones of science
and community. Scientific naturalism became the new builder of
absolutes and sustainer of realities, and scientific naturalism depended
on its postulate of extrinsic relations between discrete objects: the
public reality. In a profound sense science was a new puritanism,
dividing the human being into good and evil—the public (predictable), objective self (not the person one sees, but the one science
detects), and the private (unpredictable), subjective self. As the new
demonic, the private becomes the source of all devilish occurrences:
the compulsions, the obsessions, the fits—the bizarre and the eerie. In

community this demonic private self would be washed away in the blood of the lamb of the public reality. It would be made unconscious—*the* unconscious—then transformed into public reality through action. At that point the self, which science sees in behavior and the objective self which science detects behind behavior, will become one. The real and the phenomenal will merge. Here, on the plane of the public reality, community and science become twin ideals. The Real Miss Beauchamp would emerge in a land where purity means clarity. Hall had made himself the theologian of Miss Beauchamp's resurrection and apotheosis.

Hall was doing his bit to consummate what had been in the works in scientific circles since Galileo and his "secondary qualities," the identification of all that is in flux, all that defies anticipation, all that cannot be quantified, with the private and with the subjective. Thus, Hall explained away the whole phenomenal world (the side of sensation) as a lower reality. Mental illness became the condition of living in that realm.

But Hall did not stop at the point represented by traditional English empiricism, where the object (the tree) has its subjective representation (our idea of the tree), and the subject and object coexist in an uneasy truce. Like James, he pushed to the non-Cartesian dualism. For James the situation of having two mutually exclusive worlds existing together was but a resting place before going on to a neutral monism where there is neither subject nor object. But to achieve this, James opted out of the dialectic of objectification by forsaking his pursuit of perceptual control. For Hall the resting place became a prison, a house of horrors wherein one is both dream and object, an adolescent, and a somnambulist. He could not opt out of the dialectic by taking James's way because the pursuit of perceptual control was his life. So he imagined rising *above* it: give up the self that is both dream and object by losing oneself in community, the higher. Sally—the source of the odd and unpredictable—will have been banished.

Hall's community was social theory's analogue of the neuro-physiological higher levels—the realm of the rational. But it was something more, also: the ideological statement of Prince's doctor-patient relationship. In it one takes both sides of that relation, the dominance of the doctor and the submission of the patient. The people who espoused this ideology had the effrontery to call others schizophrenic.

In the *Varieties of Religious Experience,* James asked science to listen to the private and the individual. He hoped to save religious experience from being stigmatized as aberrant behavior. He hoped also to deter science from the rigid determinism that polarizes the possibilities of reality into total structure or total unstructure. His scheme required that the object not be seen as a discrete entity defined separately from its relations in the stream. He was asking the scientist to relinquish his privileged position as truth-giver and to give equal time to the religious person. The scientist's reality—the public reality—would be lowered to the level of private experiencing.

If one was after certainty, James's way was objectionable on all counts. And, besides that, to some there seemed a better way to save religion—its elevation to the level of science by eliminating private experience from its corpus and by making the argument that religion operates on the high ground of the public reality. One could equate religion with order and control, that is, with science itself.

The psychology of religion movement began in America as an attempt to make religion respectable by making it a science. Hall's role in this was as important as it was anti-Jamesian. As usual, he sought to control the movement—by guiding his own Clark University students into it, by founding and editing *The American Journal of Religious Psychology and Education* (from 1904), and with his thunderous two-volume *Jesus the Christ in the Light of Psychology* (1917). But others were reacting to James also. Scholars at the University of Chicago, Columbia, and Harvard reacted. And, at Harvard two of James's own students, Ralph Barton Perry and Edwin B. Holt, guided the reaction into a philosophical movement called the New Realism, joining hands with the new psychology called behaviorism. Both groups—the psychologists of religion and the New Realists—took as their point of departure the intermediate stage of James's development (the non-Cartesian dualism), with important consequences for American Freudianism. Through them, Hall's idea of community gained philosophical respectability.

When, in 1891, Charles Francis Adams wrote that the "morbid excitement" of religious revivals was a species of insanity, and when John McMaster, in his 1885 *History of the People of the United States,*[32] described an early revival in terms of "nervous and hysterical disorders," those historians were rehearsing an academic tradition that reached back to an elitist reaction against the Great Awakening in the 1740s.[33] What was new in Hall's 1881 public lectures at Harvard was his idea that religious conversion is an adolescent phenomenon.[34] He brought religious excitement into the context of his later "genetic" psychology and got ready to fit it into the context of cultural evolution.

In an early Clark University publication, Arthur Daniels wrote that anthropology is "the pedagogical root and very lifespring of theology."[35] The anthropology Hall's group had in mind was somewhat that of German *Volkerpsychologie*, but principally that of English evolutionary ethnology: Edward Tylor, Andrew Lang, and, the master, James George Frazer of *The Golden Bough* fame. In his *Primitive Culture*, Tylor wrote that ancient man "has never learned to make that rigid distinction between subjective and objective, between imagination and reality" and that preliterate men could "scarcely distinguish between their dreams and their waking thoughts."[36] Hall was all ears.

The historical enquiry into the roots of anthropological thought on these matters has yet to be made. Perhaps the ethnologists' assumption that ancient man had no ability to abstract or generalize relied on missionaries' failures to convert native peoples to monotheism. On the other hand, Frank Manuel (*The Eighteenth Century Confronts the Gods*) has shown that the philosophes impugned the preliterate mind in order to enhance that of their own age. Their ancient man was prelogical and prescientific, a man living in a world of immediacy and concreteness. Nineteenth-century *Volkerpsychologie* advanced a similar thesis through its roots in romanticism. Thus we find Max Müller in his 1889 Gifford Lectures on *Natural Religion* arguing that language evolves in its complexity and generalizing powers as civilization advances.[37]

To the evolutionary ethnologists, then, preliterate man was the childhood of the race; but the English gave the idea a twist of their own in the statement by Tylor and Lang: "it becomes possible to realize a usual state of the imagination among ancient and savage peoples, intermediate between the conditions of a healthy prosaic modern citizen and a raving fanatic or a patient in a fever ward."[38] Again, Hall was all ears.

The exceptional religious states described by James and observed by others became, in Hall's anthropology, the rise of the savage dream. James Leuba, one of the Hall group, responded to *Varieties* with this: "Truly the new beatitude is a hard saying: 'Blessed are the intoxicated, for to them the kingdom of the spirit is revealed.'" He described James as giving religious significance to "mystical, insane and drunken dreams," and added: "The running rats and twining snakes of delirium tremens would stand unimpeachable together with the doctrinal beliefs and hallucinations of saints and the dreams of sleeping life."[39] Josiah Morse, another Hall pupil, was similarly vexed. The *Varieties* should have been entitled "Varieties of Abnormal Religious Experience," since all of James's examples were cases for the asylum. Both men echoed Hall's premises: Morse spoke of the "naive and childish mind of primitive man" for whom the "mysterious is always deified," and Leuba explained: "Religious faith and asexual love are hardly to be found in the lower civilizations. They are late products of human development, the existence of which is conditioned by higher powers of generalization."[40]

Antipathy toward James was not universal. Edwin Starbuck and James Bissett Pratt liked the *Varieties*, yet they too were hooked on English ethnology. In 1897, leaning on Hegel and on Frederich Schleiermacher one of Hall's favorite philosophers, Starbuck had portrayed the adolescent falling out of childhood innocence of received custom into the despond of self-consciousness. The adolescent is shocked out of childhood by the voice of the racial past, the "unconscious." Starbuck contended that religious enthusiasm speaks to this state, drawing the youth further along the dread road of withdrawal. Quite different is the true religious experience, which pulls the individual out of his self-consciousness and puts him into harmonious submission to God and human institutions.[41] Starbuck, too, was in the camp of Hall.

Through his own writings and those of his best students (that is, Leuba, and Starbuck), Hall stamped the psychology of religion movement with his thinking. The Hegelian-Schleiermacherian theme of fall from innocence and return to community became the compelling one. Pratt used it in his *Psychology of Religious Belief* (1908), though he wrote that above all "I am indebted to the assistance and inspiration of Professor William James." Pratt made the Jamesian "subliminal" the "inheritor of our past and forms what might be called a feeling memory."

Through it one becomes united to the race, and through the race to the cosmos. The primitive mind, like the child's, Pratt explained, was one of simple faith and extreme credulity. Moreover, all "anthropologists agree that primitive man makes comparatively little distinction between the dream state and the waking perception, so far as their relative reality is concerned." Primitive man's mentality is "fantastic" and "bizarre," "verging on the abnormal or the positively insane." He cited Tylor, Müller, and also Hall's *Adolescence* as his sources, but he turned to Starbuck to support his conclusions about the religious awakening. The result was completely un-Jamesian: the subliminal becomes a racial consciousness that rescues the self-conscious, alienated adolescent with one of two results: either the calm union with the universe or the pathological state of diseased excitability characteristic of American revivalism.[42]

On the other hand, Pratt argued that religion must be divorced from science.[43] In taking this position, derived from James's idea that true religion is a private experience, Pratt was the exception. But his example is instructive, nevertheless. He accepted most private experiences, but not those sorts James thought were the crucial proofs of divine origin—the "fantastic" and the "bizarre." In trying to reconcile science with chance, and thus with religion, James had left behind even the faithful Pratt.

The concept of adolescence drew to it all the late-nineteenth-century feelings of estrangement. It spoke with special urgency to the emerging professional intellectual and found a significant place in his social theory. In *Adolescence*, Hall gave the psychology of religion movement its central motif by characterizing man's march through the ages as steps from primitive unself-consciousness through alienation and individualism into the higher selfhood of community. Similarly, James's description of the fading self—the self felt in the sting of immediate experience but which fades in self-consciousness—was becoming a reality for the professional. For George Albert Coe of Columbia University, Hall's coeditor on the *American Journal of Education*, and for Edward Ames, of the University of Chicago, the fading self was the point of departure.

Coe and Ames subtly but crucially shifted ground from Hall toward the Jamesian-derived functionalism of Chicago's J. R. Angell. They felt bound to accept the stream as the true description of immediate experience, but they had no desire to relate to such an evershifting and unpredictable world and saw in the *Principles* a way towards treating the self, for example, as substantial and organized. James described an empirical "Me" that comes into existence as an object of reflection. It exists as a series of behaviors that get tied together in an enduring entity (and felt to be "mine") by the feelings of warmth and intimacy associated with them.[44] For James, the "empirical Me" was merely functionally real, never to rise above the arbitrariness of any other objectified portion of the stream to emerge as an ontological fact. But the Chicago School, and particularly the philosopher-psychologist George Herbert Mead, found a way to raise the level of the reality of the me—through the idea of *emergence*.

Mead identified the empirical Me with James's "social self" (defined by the way we perceive others perceiving us) and united that idea with the notion (like Hall's) that society is an emergent. In that case, the empirical Me becomes an emergent along with the society that creates it. Mead passed the function of self-reflectivity (the function of creating the empirical Me) over to society. He argued that it is due to the fact that we see ourselves through the eyes of others (via the complexities of symbolic interaction) that we emerge out of the nonreflective (lower) level of immediate experiencing. Society has this power of conferring a self (along with a mind and reflective thought) upon one.[45] Hall and Mead were unlike in most ways, but their end result was a concept of society that, in endowing one with selfhood, had the functions of a divinity.

Coe and Ames, with others in the psychology of religion, took over these ideas and easily fit them into a religious context.[46] Convinced as he was by James, Coe simply stood James on his head.[47] The stream is truly reality, but it is an experiencing by the child and the savage from which modern civilization rescues the adult. Taking from Mead the idea that the power of reflection resides in the collectivity (in effect, society *is* the conscious ego), Coe could argue that the infant emerges from the stream into the subject-object perceptual orientation as he or she becomes socialized.[48] This notion was to become standard for American psychiatry. The stream (neutral monism) was conceded to be real enough for the infant (infant narcissism) but the subject-object dualism becomes the reality for the adult because socialization is emergence. The idea of emergence conveniently solved the problem of realities: both the infant's stream and the adult's dualism are real.

This curious metaphysics smacked strongly of Hall's, in which there was one reality for perception (unstructured sensation), another for conception (the structured world of science). The problem was the same — entrapment in the non-Cartesian world. In detaching himself from his own ideas, feelings, and behavior, the professional made an object of himself, yet he yearned to return to a land beyond self-objectification and role playing. He dreamed of spontaneity, of lost childhood. But Sally stood on the far side of the intervening gulf called adolescence. The adolescent was Mead's "I," living a nonsubject-object, dream-like existence. It was the self that is exposed when the "me" disintegrates before ambiguity, the self that psychiatry would soon learn to call "the unconscious."

Coe urged a multifaceted thesis: one becomes truly socialized in the religious conversion experience; group perception is scientific perception because it is public; the "empirical Me" that emerges in the group is the real, scientific self. "Conversion," he wrote, "is a step in the creation of a self — the actual coming-to-be of a self. . . . In conversion the pronoun 'my' acquires meaning that it did not have before; mere drifting, mere impulse, are checked." Coe was saying that in religious conversion I enter community and suddenly discover the real, public me, the me that is object in the eyes of others. One steps out of the dream into the clear light of the public reality: "Conversion is generally, perhaps always, a step in the creation of society. . . . A distinction is made between a lower illusory self and a higher or valid self." Emergence into community, and into mental health, becomes a religious event. Thus Coe reversed James. God is not to be found in the privacy of the subliminal: "That any Christian theologian should regard it as a gain for religion when men look for God in the dim, outlying regions of consciousness rather than at the focal points called 'I' and 'thou' is rather surprising."[49] God is community: "I" and "thou." Clearly, James was no Christian theologian.

Like James and Hall before him, Coe was disturbed by the fading self. But again Coe turned James around. The self is not in the "sting," but in the eyes of others:

> When, therefore, the Brahmin thinks to discover the real
> world by introversion, ignoring the social reality that is immedi-

ately before him, he excludes from his data the only experience
that can sustain his sense of his own reality. . . . As social participation in one another's experiences is the only corrective for
dreams, so also it is the only sure bridge between the abstracta
of reflection and the concrete world order. . . . Science knows no
private fact, no unshared truth. It is in society that real objectivity
arises and has meaning.[50]

Coe was working out the non-Cartesian dualism. The world of the
purely subjective has become the lower; the world where everything,
including the self, is object — the world defined by the public reality — has
become the higher.

Ames began, like Coe, from the Jamesian premise that the individual's
reality is the stream, and then went on to urge that it is by emergence
out of the stream into the group that one attains to the higher, self-
reflecting consciousness and the subject-object perceptual orientation.
In his account, once civilization reaches the higher level of community,
private experience "becomes abnormal and inconsequential . . .
pathological and despicable." At the higher level, religion is the "deepest
phase of the social consciousness," and "nonreligious persons are
accordingly those who fail to enter vitally into a world of social
activities and feelings." But, warned Ames, there are those incapable
of so sharing — those like idiots, paupers, hysterics, and, generally, the
insane.[51]

Ames closed the door of community to those who would retain
subjective feelings of selfhood. He brought forward an idea destined
to be a powerful factor in American psychiatry, an idea derived from
James's definition of "mind" as the whole person in action: the
doctrine of the *act*. Angell of Chicago and others turned the idea into
a particular brand of functionalism. "Mind" becomes an objective
thing — that is, behavior. It is thus thrust into the public reality. Now
science can study the mind as it ascends upwards towards community; science becomes theology, tracing the soul's ascent towards
salvation. "The psychology of religious experience," Ames wrote,
"becomes conditioning science for the various branches of theology,
or rather, it is the science which in its developed forms becomes the
theology or the philosophy of religion."[52] The doxological approach
to science was thus revived and made ready for twentieth-century

American psychiatry. Incredibly, it was revived by enshrining pure objectivity and a world purely object.

The psychology of religion aspired to be a new theology. Its god was community, its holy spirit, science. Its hell was the isolated individual (collectively, mass man), inescapably locked into his private world. Its heaven was the attainment of the sense of selfhood—a self made substantial through the eyes of others. There was the self and world of pure subjectivity—that of the savage, the adolescent, and the dream. Only by emerging into community does one realize that that world is an illusion, that there is only one reality—the public. Hall, Mead, the psychologists of religion, they all worked from a non-Cartesian base that envisioned two side-by-side worlds. By labeling one a savage, adolescent, or insane dream, it seemed possible to exorcise it, leaving for sane contemplation a world only of concrete, substantial, and real objects. Thus the higher-lower doctrine lived on to become a social philosophy and an ideology for the middle-class professional.

The new perceptual orientation, formalized in psychology as functionalism and the genetic approach to the higher-lower doctrine, needed (one might say) to be grounded in formal philosophy. The need was met by the New Realism, representing some of America's leading academic philosophers in the 1920s. Its prominence was seriously contested only by pragmatism. The latter placed more emphasis on the practical and on social action, while the New Realism emphasized the reality of logical relations. Pragmatism went further towards breaking with atomism with its discrete objects and extrinsic relations. Both were strongly influenced by James, but both attempted to fit neutral monism into the scheme of the non-Cartesian world.

Because the New Realists appreciated Freud, they influenced American psychiatry. Because the pragmatists ignored Freud, psychiatry ignored them. This fact has determined my decision to deal with the New Realists. I have selected two Harvard professors who were once students of James: Ralph Barton Perry and Edwin B. Holt.

In 1912, six American philosophers banded together to produce a manifesto and exposition, *The New Realism*.[53] That same year, Perry, one of the six, independently explored contemporary philosophical themes in order to highlight the new philosophy. Jamesian in its neutral monism, it nevertheless leaned heavily on the teachings of Bertrand Russell and G. E. Moore in England.

What worried Perry about James's pure experience was that it seemed not to allow for the independent existence of entities outside one's private experiencing.[54] Does a tree, a house, or another person exist outside my experience? Of course they do, and nobody doubts it; but from Perry's point of view, James's radical empiricism denied it. The stream, wherein things are experienced immediately with no separation between subject and object, seemed to Perry a true description of private experience only. Here again, in philosophy, as in psychology, we find the central reaction to have been directed against the idea of private reality.

Dewey and pragmatism made experience public by handing it over to the agency of community through the instrument of science. Perry refused to take that route because his real world had to be independent not only of the individual but also of society.[55] He adopted instead a position he called "epistemological monism": our idea of a tree is, as James said, the tree, not some subjective image of the tree. The entities Perry described were neither mental nor material, they were neutral, becoming one or the other only in retrospection. To this point, he had not gotten beyond James. The problem was to sustain an argument that such neutral entities do exist when not experienced. He might have gone another step with James and looked for the substantiality of such entities in their potential—the "more"—but this opened up James's wild world of chance, and Perry was having none of it. Instead he looked to the unperturbable world being built by Russell out of logic.

Perry was blocked from making his entities (his trees, people, telephones) substantial by his assertion that they are neither mind nor matter. But if not substantial, in what sense might they be real? He looked to the relations between objects—they could be measured, thus their public reality was assured. By analyzing an entity into mass, weight, dimensions, force, energy, and so forth, one realizes that all these things are measurable. They must themselves be relations extrinsic to the entity. What then remains of the entity, once its physical properties are analyzed into relations? Only the logical concept and/or the mathematical variable, nothing more. But nothing less, also. Logical or mathematical entities conform nicely to the rule of neutral monism—not mind, not matter, and they transcend individual (and social) consciousness. They and their relations thus, said Perry, constitute reality. Further, one sees that logic and/or mathematics govern that reality because the concepts or variables together with their relations constitute the laws discovered by science. One notes that these laws are public.[56] Thus, like Hall, the New Realists chose to begin with the billiard-ball world and work from there to absolute order at the expense of chance and the sting of private experience.

But what of the human being? Was there any place for him or her in the New Realism? Only for his objective, public side. For Perry and Holt there was no other side, no valid private experiencing lying outside the public realm. None. Looked at one way, the New Realists believed the individual to be just like any other entity—a mathematical construct. All the qualities an individual might possess can be reduced to extrinsic relations: his mind is simply his behavior. This conclusion led Holt, in 1915, to elaborate a philosophical and psychological basis of behaviorism.[57] We again arrive at the functionalism of Angell.

The same conclusions could be reached from other directions. Perry noted that James's theory of emotion enables us to ignore subjective words like "feeling."[58] He and Holt took James's chapter on the "Consciousness of Self," in which the entire self was reduced to objective dimensions, as the whole show. The New Realists followed Hall in building on one side of the early James and in entrapping themselves in the non-Cartesian dualism. Fearing Dionysius, they entrusted the world to Apollo.

Freud's ideas (with the blood and guts drained) fit nicely into the New Realist scheme. In *The Freudian Wish and Its Place in Ethics* (1915), Holt argued that Freud had revolutionized psychology by shifting its interest from sensation (subjective and private) to the wish, that is, to behavior (objective and public). Freud's "unconscious wish" is merely a "course of action" that the (human) organism is programmed to carry out.[59] The wish becomes objectified in the act. Holt landed for a moment in the world of Watsonian behaviorism, but quickly sped away into the land of doxological science by introducing his notion of (Aristotelian) "form." It is in action that one fulfills one's form, transforming the potential into the actual. The concept of form—so reminiscent of Thomas Laycock's nineteenth-century handling of reflex arc theory—gave Holt the right to talk about emergence out of false subjectivity into objective reality. "Form" is selfhood, the seed burst into flower. It is Miss Beauchamp romping forth into the sunshine of womanhood—as a construct in mathematical logic.

In suppressing certain wishes, said Holt, in refusing to carry them into action, a person becomes sick—mentally ill. The person who has repressed his wishes is lower level, individualistic, morbidly subjective. The sane person has transformed inner potential into observable behavior. He stands objectified in the spotlight of the public reality. He has become ethical, also!

> For Freud's "wish" is precisely that thing which in my defini-
> tion of behavior I call "function"; it is that motor set of the
> organism which . . . if unopposed, actuates the organism to overt
> behavior. . . . The evil resulting from thwarted integration is
> "suppression"—where one motor set becomes organically op-
> posed to another, the two are dissociated and the personality is
> split. . . . The sane man is the man who (however limited the
> scope of his behavior) has no such suppression incorporated in
> him. The wise man must be sane, and must have scope as well.
> A further and important conclusion . . . is that only the sane
> man is good and only the sane man is free.[60]

Holt tells us that the "neutral stuff" composing reality is the logical and mathematical concepts that are the universe and that are combined into laws, and "propositions."[61] He tells us that one's self, soul, or form is such a proposition generating its own development—form emerging in action.[62] The world of logical form was his ideal community. In it individuals exist as forms, logical propositions tied into the universe of mathematical logic. But, unbidden, evil has entered the world; the harmony of logical propositions has not been realized. As we nurse along those wishes that oppose our forms—those impulsions, compulsions, rages, fears—we are random, and in our randomness, sick and evil.[63] Holt's doxological behaviorism was a normative science: that which is (logically) necessary describes the realm of form, thus the good. That which defies behaviorist description (because subjective and outside observation) is random and evil.

We watch the rise of the professional philosopher. All that is real is rational because nothing stands outside the lawfulness of science. Where there is a stimulus, there is a predictable response, and it is by voluntarily entering this web of lawful relations that one's self becomes real. One becomes real (as a self) through the act, and thus predictable. The New Realism put a seal of approval on the mental health community. Its ideas would be revised and updated by modern system theory, but not essentially changed.

It is not through the passions that we discover our reality, not through the impulses that hurl a substantial body against a substantial world with a resounding crack. It is not through the lusts that set the body aflame, nor through the heartbreak that convulses the soul, that one discovers himself. It is through their controlled elimination that one becomes real as a self — if that self is a professional philosopher's role-playing selfhood.

Some pages back, I quoted Hall to the effect that "Thrice happy is he who is so wisely trained that he comes to believe he believes what his soul deeply does believe, to say what he feels and feel what he really does feel." He who cannot feel what he feels or believe what he deeply believes is ready for the new philosophy. Holt described Morton Prince as not only his revered friend but as his counsellor.[64] Prince created the Real Miss Beauchamp, Holt found her a home.

5

THE AMERICANIZATION
OF FREUDIANISM AND
SCHIZOPHRENIA

It is now time to deal with the American Freudians. We are done with the genteel and their attempts to shore up the faltering genteel faith. Our subject becomes the middle-class professionals. The agony of role and ideological redefinition was not theirs. The professionals were trained for their status from the outset of their careers, having ridden into that status on the mighty shoulders of the higher-lower doctrine. That doctrine was their mother's milk; the mental health community was their bread and butter.

The historical function of the psychiatric professional was, in part, to bring mental health liberalism into the asylums, the clinics, the universities, and the government agencies. But the process of institutionalization is not my subject, for I am on the trail of the dialectic. The dialectic was embodied in the doctor-patient relation — an area of middle-class professionalism — and mental health liberalism was the professional's ideological affirmation. But so long as the struggle for perceptual control continues and generates its residue of unstructure, the dialectic remains in motion. The doctor-patient relation was therefore quite unstable, as was its ideological embodiment. In the American Freudian we will see the professional and his commitment to the mental health ideal, but we will also notice the fragility of his situation.

As I speak of the American Freudians, I will keep my eye fixed on the higher-lower doctrine, for those who take Freudianism as new and revolutionary mistake appearance for essence. The Freudian unconscious was the Jacksonian lower with the split-off somnambulist added.

Freud attempted to analyze the dream. His was the great project of bringing the residue under control. The pursuit of structure, which had generated the residue in the first place, was now, with Freud, to be pushed further—into the residue itself. It was a grand, gallant, and self-defeating undertaking, this chase after the will-o'-the-wisp of perceptual control that was busy generating its opposite. Still, it had to be done—the psychotherapists had to make the attempt to find structure in schizophrenia—first, because the undertaking was at the heart of the American Freudian enterprise, despite the fact that Freud himself backed off from the schizophrenic, second, because schizophrenia and psychiatric theory in America had become mutually dependent sets of doctrines, two sides of the same coin. Each required the support of the other. As the area of perceived unstructure inevitably grew, the American Freudian edifice began to totter and fall, bringing down the higher-lower doctrine with it.

Until the turn of the century, American medicine was forced to couch the higher-lower doctrine in the languages of neurology and anthropology. Freud's 1900 *Interpretation of Dreams* changed that. With its publication, psychiatric language was no longer limited to the horizontal, multiple-personality approach. The great book was a liberating event, but it was fateful also. So long as it had been restricted to Prince's approach, psychiatry could stabilize the doctor-patient relationship; the unconscious could be killed, as Prince had dealt with Sally by the practice of suggesting away the patient's pains and unwanted thoughts. But with his ear tuned to the higher-lower doctrine, Freud concluded that beneath consciousness there lurks an agency that cannot be so easily wished away.

Before the onus for the ensuing events be placed too heavily on Freud's shoulders, however, it should be stressed that his great appeal to American psychiatry rested on his use of the higher-lower doctrine. Americans were Jacksonians first, Freudians second. It will be wise to get the Jacksonian element in Freud into perspective before moving on to the Americans.[1]

In the late 1880s, still very much the experimental neurophysiologist, Freud turned his attention to the problem of speech disorders—aphasia. The accepted explanation, first defined by Carl Wernicke, held that either the auditory center, the speech motor center, or the associating fibers between them get destroyed causing word deafness, speechlessness, and the like. But because in most cases these mal-functions happen only in degrees, Freud decided that the Wernicke explanation lacked plausibility. If there are varying degrees of distur-bance, there cannot be the absolute loss of one or another function demanded by the Wernicke model.[2]

Where to turn for a new model? Wernicke's was based squarely on the physiology Freud had been trained in—Meynert's. Because of a long-smoldering feud, breaking with Meynert was not Freud's prob-lem. Besides, new anatomical discoveries were disproving Meynert in crucial ways. Meynert held the cortex to be like an octopus sending its nervous tentacles outward throughout the body; sensory impressions anywhere in the periphery of this structure are sent directly back to cortical centers—visual, auditory, tactile, and so forth—there to be associated together into wholes that faithfully reproduce objects in the world. Freud objected that the scheme no longer explained the known facts: the number of fibers (nerves) ascending the spinal cord to the cortex is but a small fraction of the number going to the cord from around the body. Direct representation in the cortex of each sensory (and motor) impression is thus impossible.[3]

Freud's several masters, including Charcot in France, clung tena-ciously to the Meynert scheme. It was not until he read a paper by Hughlings Jackson that he found his alternative. In his 1891 *On Aphasia* Freud described the Englishman as this "writer, on whose views I have based almost all the arguments which I have advanced in refuting the localization theory of aphasias" and further stated that "in assessing the functions of the speech apparatus under pathological conditions we are adopting as a guiding principle Hughlings Jackson's doctrine that all these modes of reaction represent instances of functional retrogression (dis-evolution) of a highly organized apparatus, and therefore correspond to earlier states of its functional development."[4]

Hughlings Jackson's level theory precisely met the objection that not all sense impressions can possibly get to the cortex and be associated together at that level. He described a process wherein the integration of impressions into ideas is a gradual one beginning at lower levels and reaching completion at the highest. But this ap-proach offered a conception of the mind not available to the Meynert scheme. Since each of the Jacksonian levels has an integrating function of its own—a function appropriate to some evolutionary stage—each can be thought of as having its own unique function in the organism's adaptation to the environment. The higher and the lower become functional levels, the lower ever-ready to resume autonomous functioning when the higher weakens.

The 1891 shift to Jacksonian level theory was supremely important for psychoanalysis. Meynert's scheme—followed by Charcot, Janet, and Freud's collaborator in the 1893 *Studies on Hysteria,* Joseph Breuer—held that ideas become unconscious only when they are drained of energy and thus rendered inactive.[5] Level theory opened the way for Freud to argue that unconscious ideas can be very active indeed.[6]

Jacksonian level theory said nothing about an ego, but it put Anglo-American higher-lower doctrine into Freud's hands. Armed with this tool, he could deal creatively with the ego theory inherited from Meynert. Like Hall in America, he was now in a position to bring horizontal and vertical theory into synthesis. He did this for neurophysiology in his unpublished 1895 "Project for a Scientific Psychology." In 1900 he did it again in the epochal *Interpretation of Dreams.*

Meynert had defined the ego as the totality of a person's strong, active ideas. If, for reasons of disease or energy loss, the association of ideas process fails, those ideas (and the ego) become disorganized and confused. Confusion explained both mental illness and dreams.[7]

Freud was able to cast the ego in a new light, as constantly using its energies to ward off very powerful, unconscious wishes.[8] The more the ego was forced to fend against the unconscious wishes, the more drained and weakened its condition—this was Freud's expression of the self-control trap.

In 1895 Freud, in physiological and mechanistic terms, described how certain infantile wishes get painfully charged with an endogenous excitation that must be somehow discharged. The nervous system acts to rechannel excitation into new paths when those early wishes become inappropriate. Paths of discharge appropriate to adult behavior are gradually found. The ego is the unified totality of these functioning paths. However, it may be the case that appropriate paths will not be discovered. Excitation may then be discharged into nonfunctional but socially innocuous paths, such as obsessional ideas and hysterical compulsions. Still, the excitation accumulates and demands discharge. The obsessions or other symptoms grow stronger and even overwhelming.[9] Freud had found a way to express the emergence of a second, obsessional personality, which drains energies from the ego as the ego struggles to disarm those infantile wishes that themselves constitute a primal, archaic personality.[10]

The *Interpretation of Dreams* was, in important ways, a restatement of results obtained in the "Project." The dream, or dream-work, performs much the same function as the obsessions and compulsions of waking life.[11] Sleep is described as a relaxation of the ego-organization from the day's battles. Dream-work, at once expressing and disguising the primal wishes (the latent dream) makes possible the relaxation of the ego's guard.[12]

With the *Interpretation of Dreams* in print, it became possible for the Americans to personify Freud's infantile wishes as the savage of the higher-lower doctrine and, following Carl Jung, to describe schizophrenia as the savage dream. Moreover, Freud's work made it possible to hope that the schizophrenic might be helped through psychoanalytic techniques. The *Interpretation of Dreams* revealed the key to decoding the (manifest) dream and laying bare the sources of illness in the infantile wishes beneath. Dreams are not chaotic, they are organized by the laws of association, and, more specifically, they are disguises of the repressed material.[13] It becomes possible to see the dream as a code to be broken. Beneath waking consciousness lies the manifest dream, beneath that, the latent dream, and beneath that, the enraged infant.

In nineteenth-century higher-lower doctrine, the lower represented chaotic and uncontrollable impulse—the "savage." Freud brought order in the analyzable, objectifiable dream. But he gave psychiatry a theoretical system in which probing the dream unearths a deeper chaos. In 1933 he described the "id" in these terms: "the dark, inaccessible part of our personality...we approach the id with analogies: we call it chaos, a cauldron full of seething excitations.... It is filled with energy reaching it from the instincts, but it has no organization."[14]

Freud gave psychiatry its synthesis between the vertical and the horizontal and thereby gave it a language for psychic processes. He gave it, too, its great hope of bringing order to the residue. But his legacy was ambiguous. Psychoanalysis is an instrument for revealing order, an order grounded in the world's presumed mechanistic constitution. But somehow, when probed to its ground, this mechanistic order can only be described as disorder and unremitting chaos.

By putting the vertical and horizontal constructs into synthesis, Freud enabled the perception of the schizophrenic to get its formulation. I have in mind the American schizophrenic, not the version advanced by Eugen Bleuler in his 1911 *Dementia Praecox, or, the Group of Schizophrenias*, which (following Jung) gave the malady its name. Bleuler wrote in the tradition of Janet, Kraepelin, and Meynert — the association and splitting of ideas school — and lacked the Anglo-American edition of the higher-lower doctrine. The American idea of the sickness was hammered out by several profoundly influential men, Adolf Meyer at the Phipps Psychiatric Clinic in Baltimore, Smith Ely Jelliffe of New York City, and William Alanson White at St. Elizabeth's in Washington, D.C., who, with their imposing circle of adherents, created an American brand of Freudianism and established the schizophrenic as its special problem.

Bleuler's schizophrenic had a mind that constantly jumped about from one thought to another without much concern for logic or coherence. He held that the victim's ideas were fragmented into any number of conscious "complexes," each clamoring for the sufferer's attention. In their 1915 textbook on nervous diseases, Jelliffe and White bought the splitting of personality idea (thus the name "schizophrenia"), but were not satisfied with Bleuler's noncommittal "complexes."[15] By schizophrenia they meant real split-off personalities. The fragmentation of ideas was to be explained in the manner of Freud's manifest dream content; the schizophrenic is living his dream, and the dream carries its own obscure meaning. "This is," as they wrote, "the field of dream formation, of phantasies, wherein things come true."[16] They understood that in describing the dream Freud had described the schizophrenic mind. In this they were simply following Jung's 1907 exposition on the *Psychology of Dementia Praecox*: "Let the dreamer walk about and act like a person awake, and we have the clinical picture of dementia praecox."[17]

Bleuler found no meaning hidden in the schizophrenic's bizarre (he used the word over thirty times) words and acts, which come "by accident."[18] With the support of Freud's dream theory, Jelliffe and White knew better. Accident does not happen; bizarre appearances

mask underlying structure; the grotesqueness of the delusional formation is the grotesqueness of the dream, for the mechanism is the
same.[19]

For all their excitement over Freud's work, the two Americans felt
he had not carried his conclusions far enough. Freud's work, and
theory, dealt mainly with the neuroses, but Jelliffe and White thought
he held the key to the psychoses.[20] They felt also that in Freud's
discussions about regression he had overlooked the phylogenetic
implications, the savage within: "regressions may lead back to lower
cultural levels so that patients show symptoms that are only understandable in terms of the psychology of more primitive peoples." The
hand of Hall and anthropology was upon them; schizophrenia was
the primitive mind at work. Further, though they had no theoretical
quarrel with Freud's notion that resistance is directed against unconscious wishes, Jelliffe and White were less concerned about interior
conflicts than the individual's withdrawal from reality, and the outside
world. They were responding to the professional's sense of isolation.
The patient they saw was withdrawing from them.

It was bold of them to build a textbook around Freud's theories in
1915. The 1900 *Interpretation of Dreams* had at first hardly been
noticed in America, much less taken seriously.[21] The first stirrings of
interest in Freud began around 1905 and 1906 in the Jelliffe's *Journal of Nervous and Mental Disease* and in Morton Prince's Boston
study circle. In 1911 A. A. Brill, the first American orthodox Freudian,
led in putting together the New York Psychoanalytic Society and the
American Psychoanalytic Association. But this was a tiny group.
Freudianism was yet to be Americanized, and that task was begun in
the Jelliffe-White textbook.

In 1912 Jelliffe and White began laying the groundwork for starting
a *Psychoanalytic Review,* and they sought the approval of G. Stanley
Hall. "In your letter," wrote White to Hall at one point, "you said you
felt that the Freudians had not . . . seen the genetic implications. I am
sure that after your talk with Dr. Jelliffe you will feel that we have the
genetic attitude towards the problem of the dream."[22]

By now we know what that "genetic attitude" was: Hall's genetic
psychology, featuring the savage and the mental-health community,
and the functionalism that was the American response to the faltering
Cartesian dualism, the functionalism that placed exteriorizing work in

the context of "emergence." In some respects, Freudian doctrine was more convenience for the Americans than fundamental and revolutionary fact. As much as Jelliffe and White admired Freud's ideas, their first allegiance was to the higher-lower doctrine. Neither man subscribed to the sort of psychoanalytic orthodoxy that made gospel of Freud's work. Though one of the most persistent of Freud's early American supporters, White insisted that the new doctrines were at best tentative.[23] His *Outlines of Psychiatry,* said to have been American psychiatry's "most fundamental" textbook between 1907 and 1936,[24] began in 1909 to graft Freudian theory onto its higher-lower doctrine base. At various times in the pages of Jelliffe's *Journal of Nervous and Mental Disease* Hughlings Jackson was "the incomparable master," a man of "transcendental genius," to whose "profound observation and speculation" we owe undying gratitude.[25] Freud basked in no such sunshine. When assailed with self-doubts, it was good to be able to fall back upon a bedrock of presumed physical fact. Replying in the late 1920s to a skepticism raging around psychiatry's inability to deal with schizophrenia, S. C. Burchell wrote that he was happy enough to link the fate of psychiatry with the solution of that illness. We are, he said, already well on our way, having in hand August Hoch's theory of the "shut-in" personality and the knowledge (a "fundamental fact") that the schizophrenic has withdrawn, has become sly and seclusive, has, in fact, regressed to the level of "myth, magic and primitive religion." This New York psychiatrist added: "This is no new idea in medicine. It was pointed out years ago by Hughlings Jackson. . . . When a higher brain center is injured, a lower and superseded but not obliterated one comes into play."[26] Little did Burchell realize how inextricably bound together his perception of the schizophrenic patient was with his Jacksonian conceptualizations.

At the time, however, there was little reason to distrust the Jacksonian paradigm. Neurophysiology was full steam ahead in supportive findings. Americans read of investigations by Englishmen Henry Head and Gordon Holmes into brain damage—the discovery of a center for the emotions and the unconscious in the lowly thalamus, the pinpointing of the intellect in the august cortex, and the strong impression that mental illness results when cortical control over the thalamus is lost.[27] Nor were the English alone in harvesting the Jacksonian crop. At Harvard, physiologist Walter Cannon was decorticating cats and finding an "archaic portion of the central nervous system" in the thalamus, where lies the center for "emotional expression."[28] Cannon spawned a line of investigation and theory destined to dominate American neurophysiology for thirty years and more. It did not occur to onlookers from the psychiatric side of the trade that myth might have crept into the sacred halls of physical fact.

In those pioneering years of American Freudianism, the strong point was that Freud's theories dovetailed with Jacksonian physiology. But Freud worked mainly with neurotics, patients whose personalities were relatively coherent. Unmodified, his theories did not speak to the American model: Hall's adolescent, hovering on the brink of psychosis, a lonely, isolated individual, standing outside community and thus outside humanity.

Every psychiatrist seems to have one (or a very few) case that becomes paradigmatic for him, just because its successful treatment seemed to shed a flood of light. For Gray it had been Miss C. For Prince it had been Miss Beauchamp and "BCA." Boston's James Jackson Putnam's paradigmatic case was published only one year short of his death in 1918. Its principle was a certain nameless New England spinster, plagued with the region's flinty exterior. Others fled her approach. She was austere and pious, isolated and lonely, possessed of a genius for asperity. When he met her, Putnam was new to psychoanalysis. He had become friendly with Freud on the latter's memorable 1909 visit to Clark University and was drawn into the tiny psychoanalytic circle by Ernest Jones. The spinster was his chance to use the new techniques. He looked for the repressed child and found it, rendering the inevitable verdict: "dissociated personality." But something still itched.

In turning to psychoanalysis, Putnam tried to put behind him his long-time love-affair with Josiah Royce's idealism. As he looked for the repressed wishes and erotic motives, the small, still voice of his former philosophy would not quiet. The spinster's hand-writing haunted his imagination. It rounded off its letters in eloquent curves. Something more artistically creative than eroticism was there in those curves. There must be two sides to the repressed child, the sensual and the creative, the autoerotic and the "affectionate, lively, sociable, pleasure-loving." He was catching glimpses of Sally. He began to speculate that children respond not just to motives of self-gratification but to stirrings of artistic and ethical ideals—the first faint perceptions of spiritual community.[29]

Putnam's admiration of Royce's philosophical idealism echoed the genteel reaction against the coarse, scientific naturalism of the nineteenth century. Though a quiet man, he found himself making charges of one-sided mechanism not only against his close friend William James, and not only against the New Realists, who were turning to behaviorism, but also, now, against his new allies, Freud and Jones. All these people, he said, leave out a " 'something' undiscoverable by reason." None of them know " 'emotion,' in the best human sense."[30] For Putnam the reality principle—the mind—without the heart was not enough; Miss Beauchamp needed Sally.

This was a hard thing, certainly. American psychiatry was heralding Freud as the lawgiver to the unconscious, the tamer of chaos, yet in its thirst for the doxological it objected to his mechanism. But Putnam crossed Freud in another way. For Freud, the great fact of mental illness was the constant pressure from threatening wishes, and the cure lay in self-understanding. For Putnam, the central fact of mental illness and of the modern consciousness was the individual's "sense of isolation, doubt and terror . . . jealousy . . . depression and despair." His theme was the same sense of incompleteness felt by James. His words expressed the cry of the fading self, the underside of the genteel mind, the vision of the abyss. Putnam's cure was to regain completeness in community.[31]

The bloodless and cerebral Roycean philosophy of the "Absolute" that guided Putnam had little appeal, even when dressed in the clothes of community. Hall's community, by contrast, attained a certain robustness in his idea of the racial drive for life and procreation. That sort of thing was meat for Smith Ely Jelliffe, a veritable dynamo of the American Freudian movement who, when he wasn't practicing his analytic techniques on Mable Dodge Luhan and converting Karl Menninger to psychoanalysis, was editing the *Journal of Nervous and Mental Disease* and coediting the *Psychoanalytic Review* with his intimate friend, White.

In his time, Jelliffe knew enthusiasm for Jung, Henry Bergson, and Alfred Korzbyski, along with a dozen lesser lights. He sprinkled his Freudianism with their insights, but always with one goal in mind: the introduction of the twin ideas of "emergence" and "reductionism" into the body of American Freudianism. He and White, with their admirers, were fortifying the doxological approach, and because of their commanding position in American psychiatry throughout the 1920s and 1930s, a version of the doxological thrived.

The Americans had long been loath to abandon man's spirituality to scientific naturalism. In their several ways, each of the men I have talked about made the human spirit his central concern. Gray introduced the "conscious ego"; Hall embodied that function in "community," or science. From Gray to Hall the tendency was to locate human spirituality in mental health, that is, in predictability. Thus when Prince uncovered Sally, he was blind to her as a creative force, and when James suggested that creativity makes its appearance in the fitful, the humbugging, and the wild, his colleagues found him dangerous. Perhaps it was Putnam's rediscovery of Sally's blithe spirit that helps account for the new note in the work of Jelliffe and White — the notion that a creative power emanates from the lower. But there was another useful tradition at hand, the vitalism picked up by Ray and his friends to explain their moral insanity doctrine. Rediscovered in the Freudian libido, vitalism still had an important role to play.

Jelliffe and White proceeded along the well-established course of trying to wrestle scientific naturalism (that is, Freudianism) into the doxological mold. It seemed possible that though mechanism gives the truth, it does not give *all* the truth. It adequately describes the automaton, and in dream theory it adequately describes dream-work. But it is not adequate to the sane person. He or she has emerged. Long before, in 1878, the French physiologist Claude Benard ended a raging debate between chemical physiologists and life force vitalists by observing that the body creates a new environment in which, while chemistry remains chemistry, different properties of the chemical elements than had hitherto been active are brought into play. Thus it could be argued that the life sciences introduce new terms; there is an "emergence." And it might also be argued that the human sciences deal with an even further emergence.

Hughlings Jackson's "higher integrative levels" could be viewed as emergent levels. Community consciousness could be viewed as an emergent beyond individual consciousness (which in community becomes the lower, the unconscious). Freud could be spiritualized by putting his idea of "sublimation" (the transformation of sexual energy into cultural pursuits) into the context of emergence, as Hall had already done. As a human science, psychiatry becomes a spiritual activity.

Jelliffe's search for the spiritual led him into the dramatic arts. In the Broadway theater he experienced powerful evidence of the libido's creative energies. *Psychoanalysis and the Drama* (1922), written with Louise Brink, directed attention to the struggle between emotion and the reality principle. Unconscious wishes are fashioned by the artist's agony into creative art. In drama we watch individualism's stubborn rebellion against community. We watch rebellion's final submission to the great life force of the race, that vast emotional life which lies beneath the far narrower rational life and is thereby largely the master of it." We see that Freud's unconscious wishes are racial energies, the forces that forge the higher unity. For Jelliffe and Brink the "immeasurable stream of energy or libido" was finding expression in community, mastering the "antisocial attitude and those lawless individual tendencies which mark it," overcoming individualism's attempts to repress and redirect the libido into "infantile and primitive conditions and modes of reaction."[32] The Jelliffe-Brink individual was a way-station for the racial libido in its passage either onward and upward towards community or downward in a plunge back into the primitive racial unconsciousness: schizophrenia and the abyss. It was Hall all over again, but with a touch of Sally.

Again, in the *Technique of Psychoanalysis* (1918), Jelliffe stated his theme:

> Libido is . . . the living vital energy, which, flowing into various forms, as Bergson has so well expressed it, may be compared to a string of pearls. The organized living forms of plants and animals are comparable to condensations at different points along the string. We term the latest crystalization man, the next, possibly . . . the true superman, the futuristic, socialistic ideal, more closely allied to the symbolic Christian ideal than any as yet reached.[33]

Freud had taught that social order is the cause of repression; the Americans taught the opposite, that social order is the condition of release. In the isolated individual, Jelliffe thought, libido or energy is so dammed up by its inability to find release in social activity (sublimation) that it must be repressed. For the Americans, individualism became the condition and the symptom of insanity. The isolated individual, the crowd man, his libido repressed, remained behind in the realm of the lower, the realm of mechanism. White expressed their idea of the libido as follows:

> We have come to conceive of the psyche as a manifestation of the great creative energy inherent in all life — as energy always stressed with possibilities for upward progress, always struggling, as Bergson would put it, to free itself from the restraints of matter — to become more and more spiritualized — in response to the all-pervading *pousée vitale*.[34]

Not very far beneath the surface of Jelliffe's thought there was always that tension to which I have been giving the images of Sally and the "Real" Miss Beauchamp: creative freedom stood over against control and predictability. There was always the hope that the tension would be resolved by the idea of emergence, and by the magic realm wherein freedom lies in order, the mental health community.

To this point, I have introduced two ways in which Freudian doctrine was readjusted to America. It had to be retooled to deal with the American vision of the lower — the schizophrenic. In a short while I will develop these themes in the thought of William Alanson White. But first I must introduce yet another readjustment that had to be made, a difficult one to conceptualize because it reaches into the perceptual dialectic itself. This was the attempt to square Freudian (and Jacksonian) doctrine with the American monistic functionalism as preached by Perry and Holt. It was the attempt to break out of the isolating subjectivity that threatened the professional by plunging into the public world of the objective, active life. It was the project of the mental health liberal's ideal community, the project of regaining one's selfhood through losing one's isolated and fading self (submission) by gaining perceptual control over the other person (dominance), and it grew out of a dualism that was not Cartesian, a dualism in which all is dream and, at the same time, all is object.

If functionalism had been taken in the sense William James intended — in the context of the neutrally monistic reality of the stream—the dichotomy between chaos and order would have been put aside as human artifacts and conceptual abstractions, and the mythical lower, as embodiment of both sides of the dichotomy, would have been eliminated. Then the philosophy of the act would not have come to embody the promise of a return to order through the elimination of chaos-producing (split-off) subjectivity (that is, the Freudian unconscious conceived as the isolated, dream-entrapped individual) nor the rise above mechanism through emergence.

A representative statement of the functionalist formula would be this one made by psychiatrist Adolf Meyer in 1916: "Action is both the foundation and the climax of mental life; talk and feeling and thinking are but a way to action, and depend for their wholesomeness on action." He further stated in 1925: "As has been said, 'The laws of mental health and of character require the completion of thought or feeling by expression in action.' Mere feeling and thought and fancy which are not brought to the test of action, to their fulfillment in action, tend to become one of the danger points of human nature."[35] The philosophy of the act became a vital part of mental health liberalism. It was a philosophy for industrial production, for reaching out to the markets of the world. It was a philosophy for professionals, for men and women for whom technical competency is uppermost.

William James was Meyer's favorite philosopher. The Swiss-born psychiatrist pounced on James's chapter on habit in the *Principles*—James at his most healthy-minded. Meyer was unaware of the philosophical distinctions between James and New Realists like his friend Frederick Woodbridge, editor of the *Journal of Philosophy, Psychology and Scientific Methods*. Consequently, Meyer had as much to do with psychiatry's rejection of the sick-souled James as did that arch-enemy of all things Jamesian, G. Stanley Hall.[36]

My use of Meyer as the spokesman for psychiatric functionalism is no accident. He was its leading advocate in America. He was also one of the two or three leading American psychiatrists between the two world wars.[37] With his friend and fellow Swiss immigrant August Hoch, he gave American psychiatry its characteristic definition of the schizophrenic—the "shutin" personality. This definition conformed to his philosophy of the act, which, he believed, supplied the dynamics of schizophrenic aetiology in a way superior to Bleuler's notions: "I thus come to describe the development of dementia praecox as being essentially a deterioration of the instincts of action."[38]

Meyer got his start along the road toward becoming an authority on schizophrenia when he took a short leave from the Worcester asylum in 1896 to study under Emil Kraepelin at Heidelberg. He brought back the new Kraepelin nosology, which separated out dementia praecox as a specific disease entity. He also brought back a tendency, shared by Bleuler, to retain the experienced world as his reality. Against the higher-lower doctrine and the multiple-personality theories, he opposed his own "organism as a whole," that is, the reality of the person who stands before us, just as we see him.

Meyer worked effectively to get the new nosology accepted — as Director of the New York State Psychiatric Institute from 1902 to 1910, he was in the position to do so — but he was upset by the Kraepelin approach just the same. He was upset, first, because of the fatalism implicit in the concept of a disease defined by the assumption that it must inevitably deteriorate into dementia; he was further upset by the concept of "disease entity" itself. Can we abstract out a group of behaviors and call them a disease without losing sight of the person?

In the best Germanic tradition, Meyer was pure scientist; slight and immaculate, shy and linguistically unapproachable, yet an inveterate rebel, he devised a psychiatry ("Psychobiology") whose lack of system was its hallmark. Systems kill the spirit; he had fled Europe in the first place in search of a science compatible with the human spirit. Thus his joy in discovering James. But somehow his Jamesian bent led him to the thing he called "mental hygiene": "With the recent change," he said in 1918, "the force of these influences [dogma and tradition] has lessened tremendously, and it is actually up to modern mental hygiene to bring back on the new basis a new respect for a new spirituality and morality and conscience."[39]

Meyer was born in a village near the city of Zurich, the son of a Zwinglian minister. Personal ambition took him to the University of Zurich, but the spiritual search took him into psychiatry. After passing the state medical exam in 1890, Meyer studied under Charcot in Paris and Hughlings Jackson in England. He succumbed to the level theory but realized it did not satisfy his spiritual quest. As all other European physiology, it left mind separate from matter and just hanging out there uselessly. With mind irrelevant, there seemed no alternative to mechanism. He wasn't buying.

Through it all, the only glimmer of light came from America in the form of an essay from the pen of Morton Prince criticizing Hughlings Jackson's psycho-physical parallelism and offering in its stead a "dual aspect" theory: mind and matter are to be thought of as two different "aspects" of the same neutral thing. That light helped in Meyer's decision to come to America in 1892. It also became the basis for his misunderstanding of James. By 1907, Meyer was confidently describing "subject" and "object" as convenient ways of talking about the same thing: "subject" when it is perceived as acting, "object" when perceived as being acted upon. But he was also being drawn by the logic of the stream of consciousness idea towards understanding the world as process: "Our concern is with the events or 'doings,' not with the beings or final essences, and therein lies the great difference between the old frame of thought and the modern one."[40]

The Jamesian bent led Meyer toward the turgid waters of nominalism. In a world of process, where everything is defined by change, disease entities could only be abstractions. Moreover, the notion that the mind functions to abstract from the flow of experience exerted a steady tug away from the level theory. In Jacksonian lore, world events are brought into the nervous system in discrete bits and pieces, not as yet even conscious. Those bits and pieces are put together into unities as they are drawn up the steps of the integrating levels. Somewhere along the line those unities become conscious. But if, on the contrary, the mind abstracts from a stream, events cannot come in as bits and pieces; they must come in as a flow that is subsequently divided up and pigeonholed as separate concepts. In that case, there can be no distinction between "impression" and "conscious sensation," nor between sensations coming in from the outside world and from within, between impression and emotion.

For a time Meyer tried to bring the Jacksonian level theory into line with a world of process. An 1898 paper describing a "segmental-suprasegmental" approach was the result. The idea was to visualize the nervous system not as levels but in terms of "segments," each segment supporting a variety of functions, each segment entering into new combinations with others according to the function being served at the moment. He argued that each of the functional units finds its integration through some suprasegmental organ (for example, the cerebellum unites and coordinates all segmental mechanisms relating to the appreciation and coordination of equilibrium). In two subsequent papers (1906, 1907) Meyer abandoned the distinction between "impression," "sensation," and "idea." In a "dynamic psychology," he said, we do not concern ourselves with a "sharp division of sensation, idea, emotion."[41] By 1907 he had come all the way over to James. "All we know," he wrote, "is that a person as a whole sees, as part of that unit which we can also designate as the stream of consciousness, and subdivide into functional subunits or mental complexes."[42]

However much Meyer was a Jamesian at heart by that time, he still remained entranced by the dual aspect theory. It was unfortunate. In his attempt to break the chains of the Cartesian dualism, Meyer fell prey to an explanation that doubled the world. As a result, his philosophy of the act was conceived not in the Jamesian sense of passing from the subject-object alienation to the sting of immediacy but in the sense of passing out of subjective entrapment into objective action. Whatever his personal inclinations, his philosophy lent itself to the uses of mental-health liberalism.

In Meyer's scheme for the nervous system, the functional interrelation of all parts was so intricate and intimate that Hughlings Jackson's levels virtually disappeared. Meyer replaced them with the doctrine of the "organism as a whole," which, like the New Realism, described "mind" as the organism's total functioning. Similar considerations had led Perry and Holt to identify mind with behavior and to align themselves with behaviorist psychology. But Meyer pulled back from that extreme. There was in his "organism as a whole" idea the tendency to view each individual in his or her infinite uniqueness. He had struggled too long to free himself from the physiologies of Europe to follow Holt in defining away the individual in favor of his external relations. Instead, he decided that the individual as such stands beyond science. In that regard, at least, he had become a true Jamesian, but it was a very personal commitment and found few followers.

In the higher-lower doctrine, articulated by Hall and systematized by Freud, American psychiatry had its class analysis and its therapeutic mission. The lower, the isolated individual, was to be drawn by therapy into the higher state of community, thereby regaining his humanity. Psychiatry found its therapeutic program in Meyer's philosophy of the act. The individual was to be drawn out of his subjective entrapment into objective existence through action. However, neurophysiology had not caught up with the non-Cartesian world of mental-health liberalism; it was still strapped by the Jacksonian level theory to the Cartesian dualism. The task of bringing level theory into the world of American functionalism still lay before psychiatry. The challenge of doing that, and doing it without losing the supportive power of the higher-lower doctrine, was accepted by Edward Kempf, medical assistant at St. Elizabeth's Hospital.

In the early 1920s Kempf's fame briefly flashed across the skies of American neuropsychiatry. In 1920 superintendent White wrote enthusiastically to Meyer of his young assistant and golfing partner: the equal of Freud, Jung, and Adler, he said. He made the assertion again in his *Outlines of Psychiatry*. Later, in Jelliffe's *Journal of Nervous and Mental Disease*, Kempf's 1920 *Psychopathology* was declared to be one of "the outstanding contributions to the study of human behavior."[43] Kempf soon left St. Elizabeth's for private practice, thereby removing himself from the Jelliffe-White-Meyer orbit and center stage. Before long, White began to forget that Kempf's ideas were not the children of his own inventive genius.

Kempf hoped to outline a neurophysiological basis for Holt's reformulation of Freudian theory. Unconscious wishes were to be seen as tendencies to act: behavioral things, physiological things, objective things. Following Charles Sherrington of England, Kempf divided the nervous system into the "autonomic" and the "projicient," assigning to the latter the handling of the exteroceptors (eyes, and so forth) and the motor side of the reflex arc. The projicient system deals with the outside world. The autonomic system handles the body's interior environment, especially the viscera. Kempf's admiration of James, Holt, and Meyer led him to argue that thought is muscular or motor. The projicient system, then, handles perception, action, and thought. He assigned emotion to the autonomic system.[44]

Kempf claimed to build on the James-Lange theory of emotion by making thought and emotion peripheral (not just of the head but of the whole body). Actually, he drastically departed from James by dividing emotion from thought and assigning separate physiological systems and functions to each. James had said that when, for instance, upon spotting a bear one runs, the emotion is in the running—that is, the organism as a whole. Kempf was saying that emotion is in the visceral response and causes the running. His point was that the projicient nervous system obeys the dictates of the autonomic system; emotion is the master; thought, the slave. He made a further functional differentiation: the unconscious is a function of the autonomic (master) system; consciousness, a function of the projicient (slave) system.[45] Sally and Miss Beauchamp had at last received their physiological correlates.

Kempf was now ready to work Freud into his system in the way prescribed by Holt. He designated the autonomic system as the life force, the real physiological person, which must be protected, fed, and given its overt expression in the projicient system. Because of its physiological needs (nourishment, sex, and so forth) the autonomic system has wishes or demands that it makes upon the projicient system (the overtly behaving person). If the projicient system were able to unhesitatingly comply, an ideal harmony would exist between wish and act. This ideal, which turns out to be Meyer's philosophy of the act, is seldom achieved; socially disapproved wishes are repressed and live on in the autonomic system as unconscious behavioral sets.[46]

Certain physiological nuances aside, this was pure Holt; but at this point Kempf became innovative. His idea of the "I" and the "not-me" was to become the backbone of Harry Stack Sullivan's psychiatry. He argued for an "I" that is a conscious sense of self, consisting of socially approved behaviors. This "I" was thus weaker or stronger by virtue of social judgment of oneself, not by virtue of nervous exhaustion or emotional trauma as had long been the doctrine. By this time in American psychiatry, community had become the higher, and its disruption the source of sickness.

Kempf's definition of selfhood reflected the American emphasis on the individual's alienation. His "not-me" consisted of those wishes that cause loss of social approval. He equated the "not-me" with the Freudian unconscious, thus making the unconscious a barometer of alienation. His schizophrenic was one whose alienation, whose not-me, has taken over from the social "I" to become the whole of the self. Loss of esteem weakens the "I," generates the "not-me"; the social self succumbs to the alien, isolated, antisocial individual. The unconscious assumes command.[47] It was a rather brilliant formulation of the central tenet of mental health liberalism. The individual, as such, is a sickness; selfhood lies in community.

Kempf sketched in a neurophysiology for the non-Cartesian perceptual orientation. His isolated individual was dual: an object and also a dream. Lacking the higher consciousness of community, he is pure physiology, but a physiology that leads an entirely subjective existence. He can regain community by turning wish into action, otherwise the physiological wish becomes idea, and idea gets repressed and unconscious. But did Kempf (or the others) really break free from the non-Cartesian dualism with their concept of community, this dream of a purely objective existence through action in which subjective space has been expunged?

It has been my thesis all along that the ideal community, as developed by Hall and the New Realists, reflected the situation achieved in the Prince-Beauchamp relation. What that relation achieved, through Miss Beauchamp's final submission, was perceptual clarity for the doctor, a renewed sense of essence. But it was an essence with a difference.

This was not an essence — a perceptual clarity — given by ancient ties of tradition or by the sharing of strong inner controls. It was not the doxological essence that was a perceptual event for tradition- and inner-directed peoples. It was a perceptual clarity achieved through objectification and required the patient's acquiescence in that objectification. The modern professional emerged as one equipped with the techniques (and the philosophy) of objectification. With the patient's acquiescence, the old subject-object perceptual orientation (not, of course, the ideal community) was regained. Without that acquiescence, the perceptual situation tumbled toward the non-Cartesian orientation. When the patient withheld submission, the doctor was drawn into perceptual disorganization (which he disguised from himself as the patient's dream). The elimination of that dream was the aim of the philosophy of the act.

The conceptual ambiguity that was to plague American psychiatry was thus set. One goal of the philosophy of the act was to set free the individual's repressed impulses in spontaneous expression — Sally. The other goal, growing out of the psychiatrist's demands for perceptual clarity, was an individual made object through responsive and predictable action—the "Real" Miss Beauchamp.

Few were more powerful in American psychiatry than William Alanson White; few more professional. Few have left a greater abundance of correspondence and manuscripts behind for the historian, but few have left less of themselves. His scrupulously impersonal letters resemble notices; his subjective life was rigorously excluded. Did he have a subjective life? If his letters tell a true tale, he did not. The man was his work, his profession.

White's life approached the functionalist ideal of emotion transformed into overt behavior before it ever gets felt. He simply left himself no time for a subjective life of any richness. Here is an incomplete summary of his activities from the time he assumed command at St. Elizabeth's in 1903. First, he assumed the full-time administration of the hospital and the concomitant appearances before Congress on matters of appropriations and defense of his administration, dealings with functionaries in the Department of the Interior, public health agencies, the Veterans Bureau, the Army, Navy, and so forth. He lectured as a professor of psychiatry at George Washington University Medical School for many years and for briefer terms at Georgetown University and the Army and Navy Medical School. He coedited the *Psychoanalytic Review* with Jelliffe and wrote innumerable book reviews. With Jelliffe, he administered the Nervous and Mental Disease Publishing Company. He wrote well over a hundred articles, sixteen books, including six editions of his and Jelliffe's nervous disease textbook and fourteen editions of his own *Outlines of Psychiatry*. He translated books from the German, gave expert testimony at trials, and served as a consultant (for example, for the Veteran's Bureau). His support was sought and received by any number of movements—child rights, criminal rights, woman's rights—and, in particular, he became a leader in the mental-hygiene movement founded by Clifford Beers and dominated by Beers's National Committee for Mental Hygiene. He actively participated in colloquia and learned society sessions beyond number and in every part of the land. He was active in the following professional associations: American Psychiatric Association (president, 1925), American Psychoanalytic Association (president, 1916, 1917), American Psychopathological Association (president, 1919, treasurer, 1916, 1917), National Committee for Mental Hygiene (Executive Committee), International Committee for Mental Hygiene (president, 1933), Chicago Institute for Psychoanalysis (advisory board), International Congress on Hygiene and Demography (1912), American Medico-Psychological Association, Congress of American Physicians and Surgeons, American Society of Religious Education (commission on vice and crime), International Congress on Tuberculosis (1908), American Institute of Criminal Law and Criminology, Social Hygiene Society, Washington, D.C. His influence and prestige may be judged accordingly.

White's theory of therapy accurately mirrored the life of the impersonal professional. In his "The Mechanisms of Transference" (1917), he argued that what a patient supremely needs is a feeling of stable objective reality and that the therapist must provide it in the person of himself. If, by becoming emotionally involved, the therapist allows the patient to become emotionally involved with him in return, the stability of the therapist as the patient's objective reality will be threatened. Therapists should be kindly but impersonal, an approach well-tailored to White's personality, but tailored as well to his functionalist philosophy, in which subjectivity and emotion are to be transformed into objective behavior. "Consciousness means virtual action," he wrote in the same article, quoting Bergson; and "the fundamental law of psychical life is the orientation of consciousness towards action." White added: "All this absolutely justifies the statement by Hall where he says: 'Epistemologically speaking, no one can know what he does not objectify.' Then, if we will also take into consideration the wish, as Holt does, as a 'motor attitude,' 'a course of action which some mechanism of the body is set to carry out,' we have a pretty complete formulation of the body as functioning by action." White's patient was to become well by objectifying himself through action. The therapist was to make this possible by objectifying himself—by becoming a stable object for the patient. Also, by this reasoning, the therapist objectifies himself through action on the patient and in this action fulfills himself as a scientist, for science is fulfilled in the act: "That perception is a process of objectification is seen when it is realized that what we perceive depends upon our particular motor set towards the object, in other words, what we proposed to do to it."[48] Like everything else in White's life, science and therapy were action.

White was committed to the functionalism of Meyer, Holt, and

Kempf, but unlike Meyer, he was just as strongly attached to the higher-lower doctrine as expressed by Hughlings Jackson and Hall. Meyer's "organism as a whole" argued against separation of intellect and emotion into centers, and White was drawn to Meyer's thesis; yet Kempf, on the authority of Holt, was doing what Meyer opposed, splitting emotion and intellect into separate nervous subsystems, and White liked *that*. His confusion made a shambles of a 1915 article on the "unconscious."

In England, physiologists Henry Head and Gordon Holmes, working in the Jacksonian tradition, directed their attention to patients with brain damage affecting the anatomical links between cortex and thalamus. They concluded that the thalamus is the center for emotion, the cortex, the center for the intellect and higher control over the emotions. White countered with the statement that there "are no such things as emotions; there is no entity to which we can apply the term intellect," the organism acts as a biological whole and all that we can say is that there is a "feeling aspect" and an "intellectual aspect" of the total behavior.[49]

He said that in all sincerity. It put him into the camp of Meyer and, through him, James. But with equal conviction he reversed himself before finishing the article. He put the intellect (consciousness of relations) in the cortex, and feelings (the unconscious) in the thalamus. This was how he offered to explain schizophrenia. "Many reactions," he wrote, "especially in praecox, are so primitive in type that we must seek their explanation, not in the individual consciousness, but in the *race consciousness* . . . savage and infantile ways of thinking."[50] The infant lives on in the thalamus, so does the savage; and savage thought is primitive in the sense of being less structured by relations; it is closer to the stream than ours, and is thus insane.

White was plunging around in the dark when in 1917 he discovered what seemed a way out. His discovery was biologist Charles Child's "The Basis of Physiological Individualism in Organisms," in the April 1916 issue of *Science*. As was his practice when in the throes of a new idea, he rushed into print.[51]

Child had been studying microscopic creatures and making deductions for the theory of evolution. He argued that when the tiny organism acts on its environment the resulting stimulus to its body establishes a physiological-chemical axis or gradient reaching back from the point of stimulation, which now becomes the "head end." The creation of a gradient of relatively enduring chemical change in the protoplasm is the beginning of structure. Gradually, over the eons, structure and the specialization of parts develop from the original gradient.[52] The point, for White, lay in the implications this idea had for a theory of emergence. Psyche, the higher, is not a thing, a substance added to matter, it is a matter of organization, and of structure. It is in the growing complexity of structure that we have the emergence and evolution of mind out of matter: "The organism," White wrote, "did not first develop as a group of organs and *then* develop a centralized control and coordination of those organs, but the development of the centralized control and coordination went along with the development of the organs." And, from what does this structure grow? What is its source? Why, the act, of course. The organism acts on the environment, the first gradient emerges, the progeny of that first organism continue to act, and their structures continue to gain in complexity. The act gives rise to emergence, to mind. Taken singly, whether it be an organ or a person, the part, taken outside of the organization which contains it, is mere matter. Mind, psyche, the higher exists in the whole.[53]

Three years later White explained that when "it comes to the more specific problem of psychogenesis, however, it is certainly good philosophy, at least, to explain the lower by the higher and not the reverse, for the higher includes the lower and not the reverse. The union of men in society is much more than the mathematical sum of the several individuals, it contains another element, namely relations which maintain between men."[54]

White's approach was an extension of Holt's brand of functionalism. In Holt's philosophy, the individual disappeared into his behavior, his external, observable relations. The relations became the reality. With a push from Child, White took the idea a step further, approaching modern structuralism. The individual (animal or person) becomes a vehicle for the continuing evolution (emergence) of structure, nothing more. Structure becomes the permanent and immortal thing; each individual sacrifices its otherwise worthless life to it. The individual dies and is forgotten; the structure lives on, ever-growing in complexity, ever-emerging into higher stages beyond mere matter. Through structure, matter becomes mind; the individual becomes community. For structure has become the life force, the *pousée vitale*, the spiritual substance that is community. The individual, White said, is an abstraction.[55]

With Child's theory in hand, White set the stage for the transformation of his and Jelliffe's vitalism into system theory. Vitalism had taken them out of mechanism into emergence. Child's Lamarckian approach had saved them from Darwinian reductionism. But system theory could not so easily dismiss Darwin. Its advent awaited a theory that would make Darwinism available to the structuralist approach, the theory of genetic coding.

Meanwhile, White remained with Jelliffe essentially a vitalist. In October 1919, Meyer wrote to White asking where he had gotten his interesting theory of symbols. White replied that he had worked it out with Jelliffe during their summer vacations together, that it was based on Schiller's theory of emergence, which made the whole the reality, the part an abstraction. White then explained that the individual is an energy transformer—racial libido is transformed into action, thus into community or structure—and symbols are to be seen as energy containers.[56] Derived from the racial past, lodged as engrams in the soma, symbols are but latent acts, analogous to Holt's "sets" (latent behavior) and, when repressed, become Freud's unconscious wishes. But in the Jelliffe-White edition, they become the racial unconscious.

White embraced Freud's idea that dream-work is a logical exercise. The dream, he wrote, "shows us the mind operating free of intellectual critique ... guided alone by feeling qualities. Are not its results quite as logical, quite as understandable, as long as we remain at the feeling level? In fact, has it not a special validity of its own quite apart from the criteria of intelligence?"[57] This was not quite what Freud had in mind. In White's statement we seem to get a touch of Sally, or perhaps of the creative child in Putnam's New England spinster. But it is not quite Sally or the creative child either, it is the racial libido at work. Jelliffe and White were trying to capture the spirit of Sally without having to cope with her as a living reality. As an individual, she remained an abstraction.

There is in each of us this creative libido. At the time it was an appealing thought. The theory of recapitulation was in the air. In the nineteenth century, the German Darwinist Ernst Haeckel had argued that "ontogony recapitulates phylogeny." Freud, leaning on English evolutionary ethnology, had generalized the idea into a psychological statement: the individual's psychological development goes through the same stages as the race's cultural evolution.[58] Hall had said as much when he broadened the higher-lower doctrine into mental-health liberalism. By the 1920s, the idea was abroad in American neurophysiology that the human brain is formed of layers that recapitulate phylogenetic brain evolution.[59] By tracing backward down the evolution of the racial libido, White thought, one can get closer to the emotional life, closer to the poetic and creative life, closer, indeed, to immediate experiencing unblocked by the veil of abstractions that the rational mind throws over the world. The earlier stages of the racial libido live on in the unconscious and thus in the schizophrenic. In 1925 White lectured on the "Language of Schizophrenia," comparing the schizophrenic to the Melanesian, who, he thought, lacks powers of abstraction and generalization: "Now regression to a childish or primitive level of this sort, which is what occurs in those conditions in which the ego is said to lose its clearness of definition [that is, schizophrenia], does not imply a disintegration in the sense of disorder but regression to a *different kind of order* or, as my friend Korzybski would say, to a *lower level of abstraction*."[60]

Who would not like to return to the enchanted world of the Melanesian? Jelliffe, certainly, would not have spurned the chance. But above all, White was a professional. The return to a world where the heart speaks as clearly as the mind would have the psychiatrist opening himself up to his patients. Were they not closer to the unconscious than he?

The psychiatrist's job was to remain an object, to give the patient a stable world to act on and thereby to transform subjective unstructure into structured behavior. This was the assumption. But just beneath that assumption lay the fear that should the patient's world become unstable, he would begin to behave erratically or to lose control. To the professional, this would signal the rise of the unconscious—not the creative libido, not the Melanesian and his enchanted world, but something quite different. The schizophrenic, when deeply regressed, gives us entirely "alien" symbolic productions. White said, "We are not able to feel ourselves into the position [he] occupies . . . we do not understand what he says."[61]

Back in the 1915 *Diseases of the Nervous System*, White had been certain that the schizophrenic's dream-mind could be analyzed. But the discovery of Albert Storch's *The Primitive Archaic Forms of Inner Experience and Thought in Schizophrenia* (1922) carried him into a different world. Storch's phenomenological exploration of schizophrenic thought disclosed it to be made up of "absolutely undifferentiated, diffuse total expressions" and forced the conclusion that the schizophrenic's "inner experiences are indefinitely bounded off, fluctuating, and undifferentiated."[62]

Through Storch, White was carried back to the non-Cartesian world of pure subjectivity and pure object. For the Schizophrenic patient, White wrote:

> There are two types of interpenetration of the self and the world; in the one the whole world may seem to be absorbed into the self, in the other the self is absorbed into the world. For the patient of the former type all objects are merely qualities of himself made concrete, emanations from himself. This view is ... akin to the mental processes of the savages. It corresponds to the "idealistic philosophy" which regards the phenomena of the world without material existence but merely as projections of the perceiving self. For the patient of the latter type the sense of being an individual is lost, the self is felt as a dependent part of the surroundings which can penetrate into his being.[63]

Thus, through White, we find American psychiatry in the 1930s thoroughly at odds with itself. Was the dream primitive poetry or was it the non-Cartesian chaos of savagery? Was Sally to be the ideal, or was it to be the "Real" Miss Beauchamp? Would the mental health community emerge from a freeing of the "racial libido," or from the philosophy of the act wherein the individual loses himself in his overt behavior and the professional achieves his perceptual clarity? Most alarmingly, the Freudian synthesis tied the Americans to an unwanted mechanism, but in trying to escape that mechanism, they were losing the individual.

By 1940 Meyer, Jelliffe, and White passed from the psychiatric scene. They had taken up the legacy of Hall and the New Realists and fused it with Freudian theory. The American brand of psychoanalysis that they developed was extremely influential. It lacked a certain visibility in the eyes of historians because it had no formal doctrine with an easily identifiable name. Orthodox Freudian psychoanalysis or its various offshoots—Jungianism, Adlerianism, Rankianism, ego psychology—have more readily captured the spotlight. Yet the influence of White and his large circle was more pervasive than any but the Freudian orthodoxy.[64] The group included many of America's foremost psychiatric professionals. It was also intimately connected with the National Committee of Mental Hygiene and through that body not only with the federal government and its programs but with the far-flung psychiatric social work movement through which it reached out into nursing, family case work, child care, delinquency, and other areas.

The impact of the mental hygiene movement, broadly defined to include child guidance, mental retardation, juvenile delinquency, and other specialties, was to impose the medical model on cases of perceived social deviance.[65] That model has come under increasing attack by behaviorists and by skeptics from within the ranks of psychiatry. But owing to the powerful influence of the White circle, the fate of that model became significantly tied to the fortunes of the higher-lower doctrine. Following World War II, the fortunes of the higher-lower doctrine (thus to an extent the fate of the medical model) would lie in the hands of the schizophrenic, who was the living embodiment of the lower. The project to rise above the non-Cartesian perceptual orientation by curing the schizophrenic was carried out in the therapeutic situation in the 1940s and 1950s. Paradoxically, the project to cure the schizophrenic served to lock psychiatry into its own alienation.

We know now how completely the American idea of schizophrenia embodied the metaphors that surrounded the much older higher-lower doctrine. Freud had brought the higher-lower doctrine into the domain of psychiatric language. We remember that Hall had been forced to use the language of anthropology to express his thoughts, but with Freud the savage, the dream, and the machine got their psychiatric symbolization as the unconscious. White and Jelliffe had then set the unconscious firmly within the context of Hall's anthropological (genetic) approach by working out the idea of emergence. Men like Kempf and Meyer played major roles in the Americanizing of Freudian thought by bringing the New Realism to bear, particularly in the philosophy of the act. Emergence was to come through action. Action was to overcome the alienated state of the isolated individual. The higher realm—community—was conceived as a state in which people are linked into a higher unity of actions; the part loses its individuality in the structure that transcends mere parts. White called upon the psychiatrist to be a stable object for the patient; but the whole idea was to get the patient to be a stable object for the psychiatrist.

Whatever his real illness, the schizophrenic in America had become the reification of the psychiatrist's felt alienation and sense of powerlessness. The schizophrenic was the machine-dream, the non-Cartesian perceptual orientation translated into metaphor. He embodied the psychiatrist's own perceptual disorganization and consequent fading sense of self. Psychiatry toyed with the idea of opening itself to the free, spontaneous expression—the Sally—of the patient. But it took the other road, the recapture of the sense of self through assuming the role of doctor. That, however, required the acquiescence of the patient and would turn out to be a doomed exercise in magic. The project to transcend the non-Cartesian perceptual orientation by creating a stable object world (community) only served, via the dialectic of objectification, to drive the psychiatrist deeper into that perceptual orientation and that alienation. In the next chapter we shall watch the dream open and swallow the psychiatrist within it.

6

PSYCHIATRY: A FADING SCIENCE

By the late 1950s, things were not well with American psychiatry. Outside the circle of Freudian orthodoxy, psychiatry no longer had access to a theory; the higher-lower doctrine was dying. Anthropology no longer tolerated savagery as a scientific concept. Psychiatry was losing in the face-to-face encounter with the schizophrenic patient.

By 1950 the most famous name in American psychiatry probably was Harry Stack Sullivan, the wayward disciple of William Alanson White. Sullivan built his theory (and reputation) on treating schizophrenic patients and fought the great fight against American psychiatry's dehumanizing mythology. He gathered around him in Washington a small force of therapists similarly endowed with insight and sensitivity who carried his fight forward after his death in 1948. Having broken with the mythology that had defined schizophrenia and sustained psychiatric theory, Sullivan tried to teach his fellows to open their ears and listen to the patient. It was utterly dangerous advice, for the mythology had been a defense against having to listen.

Sullivan tried to shift the focus of psychiatry to interpersonal relations. He knew that there are organic problems with which neurologists ought to deal. But there are problems in living. Crazy behavior should not be located in the individual; it should be looked for in the social context in which the individual finds himself.

Sullivan acknowledged his debt to White. He was Sullivan's genius, and his inspiration.[1] A 1917 graduate of the Chicago College of Medicine and Surgery, Sullivan arrived in White's hospital in 1922 as a liaison officer for the Veteran's Bureau. After a year he departed for Sheppard and Enoch Pratt Hospital in Towson, Maryland, where he was destined to create a famed experimental ward for schizophrenic patients. He had passed through St. Elizabeth's quickly, but not before being moved by White and his promising assistant Kempf.

Sullivan became the first American psychiatrist to devote himself exclusively to schizophrenic patients over an extended period of time. Why? Researchers have found nothing in his background to account for it. Something about schizophrenic patients at St. Elizabeth's and Sheppard-Pratt appealed to his deepest nature. Did he share with them a sense of loneliness and isolation? We touch again upon a tangible thread running through the history of American psychiatry.

All through his career Sullivan stressed the place of loneliness and isolation in life. He liked to argue that anyone fortunate enough to have an intimate friend in adolescence will be immune from psychosis. Did Sullivan have such a friend? Helen Swick Perry, his biographer and long-time secretary, has said that he felt himself exposed to the schizophrenic break by his childhood loneliness.[2] His friend and training analyst, Clara Thompson, wrote of his early isolation as an Irish-Catholic farm boy in Protestant central New York state and as the only surviving child of a withdrawn, shy father and semi-invalid, complaining mother.[3] He, himself, often made oblique reference to his sense of isolation:

> The third class of isolation is primarily geographical. The only preadolescent in a sparsely settled rural community is a classical example. . . . The inaccessibility of his home — and the ignorance of his family of the significant needs of this era of growth — tend to separate him from gang life, if not from having a chum. This boy always suffers a prolongation of the adolescent epoch. . . . Fantasy processes and the personification of sub-human objects are called on. Loyalty is developed to abstract ideals, more or less concretely embodied in fanciful figures. . . . The capacity for sympathy becomes peculiarly differentiated because of the elaboration of its underlying tendencies in loneliness, among fanciful objects. From this background, there may come individuals who *finally* mature a personality that stands out well above the average level of achievement, the more in that the carrier comes to integrate interpersonal situations in which he is more of a participant observer than a unit merged in unthinking

cooperation. The force of public opinion on such a personality may remain relatively unimportant. . . .

Possessed of capacity for intimacy of extraordinary depth, his experience of fraudulent folk may easily drive him into a skepticism about people that is extremely annoying to more socialized personalities.[4]

That passage was a self-portrait. Clues are strewn throughout. In adult life, for instance, he professed an unease with stories personifying animals, which suggests a concern with an earlier brush with the enticing call of fantasy. He annoyed colleagues with his quick temper; they thought him irascible and even a bit mad. Yet he was capable of the deeply sympathetic relations described, with such people as Frieda Fromm-Reichmann, Clara Thompson, and Edward Sapir. Key words appear in the quote. "Participant observer" was the phrase he used for his method of therapy. It underscores his belief that the schizophrenic patient's acts and words are meaningful to himself and bizarre only to the unsympathetic observer. It expresses, also, his belief that the schizophrenic patient and therapist can develop the healing, sympathetic relation described. Sullivan believed, and others agreed, that he had a uniquely intimate way with his patients. So did the diminutive Frieda Fromm-Reichmann. Participation in the patient's world became their hallmark, as it did with those they influenced at the Washington School of Psychiatry and related Chesnut Lodge in Rockville, Maryland. Also, the ability to achieve intimacy became Sullivan's sine qua non for mental health. His too was a psychiatry for the lonely and bewildered.

The passage above also provides hints for Sullivan's relations with White: the lonely child's attraction to the idealized adult figure. He adored White, failing to realize that his skepticism toward White's revealed truth had turned him into an unwanted apostate. Sullivan considered himself a rebel against orthodox Freudianism within the tradition set by Meyer, Jelliffe, and White. Actually, he was a rebel against White's most cherished doctrines: community as the higher, savagery as the lower. His first published paper (1924) reflected White's positions and cited White's favorite authorities: Storch, Freud, Bergson, and Russell. But the paper emphasized a point that did not fit comfortably into White's system: the humanity of the schizophrenic.

White's idea of the emergent community rested largely on the shoulders of the lower schizophrenic. Sullivan was not buying.[5]

When he wrote, "that there is any necessity for accepting the notion of phyletic regression of mind structure is not proven,"[6] Sullivan committed the ultimate heresy. The individual inherits no primitive racial consciousness into which he regresses when he retreats from the world. Using some rough-and-ready Kantianism and the Rankian birth trauma, Sullivan tried to show that the structure of adult consciousness has its roots in one's experiences in the womb and at birth. He then speculated that the schizophrenic has regressed to the womb state of consciousness, a point at which he can begin anew to organize his perceptions of the world.

Sullivan was blundering around the sacred halls of mental-health liberalism, and toes were getting mangled. Yet he never doubted White's enduring love. Sullivan, writes Perry, had an "almost overwhelming awe for William Alanson White that lived throughout Sullivan's life."[7] Certainly Sullivan's attempts in the late 1920s and early 1930s to get White's help in restructuring America's psychiatric establishment argues against any consciousness of rebellion against White. The same can be said of Sullivan's founding the William Alanson White Institute (1933) as a shelter for rebel psychiatry. But if there was a father-son relation, it existed only for Sullivan, not for White.

Late in 1922, when Sullivan was applying to Sheppard and Enoch Pratt Hospital for a job, White wrote to its superintendent, Ross McClure Chapman, that though Sullivan is a "keen, alert, somewhat witty Irishman," the young man's "facade of facetiousness" appears to cover a "considerable discontent that might perhaps express itself in alliance with other discontented spirits." White was a good judge. Sullivan's dissensions at Sheppard-Pratt became legendary. But the fact remains that White had disparaged Sullivan to a prospective employer. In the same letter White said, "I do not feel that I really know Dr. Sullivan very well," not an auspicious beginning for a father-son relation.[8] Two years later, when the National Committee for Mental Hygiene considered Sullivan's candidacy to head up a study of the inmates at Texas State Penitentiary, White killed the prospect: "I certainly should not think of picking Dr. Sullivan for the job you have in mind. I do not believe him to be a sound man to put such a job in the hands of."[9]

In the late 1920s and early 1930s American psychiatry was in transition. The American Psychiatric Association, formerly the Association of Medical Superintendents of American Institutions for the Insane, was still largely in the hands of the asylum super-intendents, such as White at St. Elizabeth's and Arthur Ruggles of Butler Hospital, Providence, Rhode Island, and the heads of the several psychopathic hospitals, such as Meyer at Phipps Clinic in Baltimore, Charles Macfie Campbell at Boston Psychopathic Hospi-tal; and Clarence Cheney, Director of the New York State Psycho-pathic Hospital. But the center of gravity was shifting to the university-associated medical schools with which these psychopathic hospitals were allied, such schools as Johns Hopkins, Columbia, Harvard, and Michigan. Emphasis was shifting from institutional care to psychiatric training.

Again, Freudian psychiatry was making it possible for some in the profession to declare independence from neurology and physiology and still suppose themselves scientific. Many wished to declare inde-pendence, but this raised the question of whether such psychiatrists must become psychoanalysts in the orthodox Freudian sense, as some of the Freudians were demanding. The emergence of the psychoanalytic institutes—in New York, in 1931, and in Chicago in 1932, with more to follow—raised the question of how the profession was to relate to these training centers. The American Psychoanalytic Association bylaws ruled that only the graduates of institutions it recognized would be certified by the association. In short, Freudian orthodoxy was moving to dominate the practice and teaching of psychiatry. In this situation the Jelliffe-White-Meyer tradition consti-tuted a widely acceptable compromise, both between neurology and psychiatry, and between Freudian and non-Freudian approaches.

An institutional problem yet remained for the White circle. Its Americanized Freudianism, with its emphasis on community as the higher, envisioned a union with the social sciences—anthropology, sociology, and social psychology—subjects presumably to be incorpo-rated into medical school curricula. Could psychiatry absorb the social sciences and remain a medical discipline? Sullivan's close friend, the anthropologist Edward Sapir, raised this question in 1932. Psychia-trists, he wrote, were finding that their medical and biological training was of no use to them in their practice, yet their longing to be accepted as medical men restrained them from turning to their natural home in the social sciences.[10]

White promoted the union of psychiatry with the social sciences in a mid-1928 speech to the Social Science Research Council (SSRC).[11] With Sullivan, he was a member of a committee appointed by the American Psychiatric Association to open relations with the SSRC. But White seemed willing to limit his interest to the delivery of one speech, while Sullivan took the idea seriously. Under the aegis of the committee (made permanent in 1929 as the Committee on Relations of Psychiatry with the Social Sciences) Sullivan organized two now famous colloquia (1928, 1929) on personality investigation, drawing together noted social scientists and psychiatrists. Believing he had the support of White, Sullivan began formulating large plans for making the union an institutional fact. Unaccountably (to him) unforeseen obstacles appeared. In August 1929, the American Psychiatric Association resolved to study the question of psychiatric education and handed the job not to Sullivan's committee but to Yale professor Edward Strecker's Committee on Medical Services.[12] Learning that White was behind this act, Sullivan talked his friend into a compromise plan, a joint investigation.[13] The upshot was the formation of a Joint Committee on Psychiatric Education in April 1930. Then, telling White he could not work with Strecker or his people,[14] Sullivan asked for aid in purging unacceptable members.[15] The undesirables soon began to withdraw. Arthur Ruggles, for example, acquiesced and stepped aside. Superintendent of Butler Hospital, president of the potent National Committee for Mental Hygiene, Ruggles was also White's colleague on the National Research Council's committee to promote psychiatric training in medical schools. With White, he stood at the pinnacle of the psychiatric establishment, actively working to bring psychiatry into medical respectability. There is no reason to suspect that Ruggles shared Sullivan's dream, nor is there reason to believe White relished undercutting his own position within the establishment.

As Sullivan worked the Joint Committee into desired shape, he mapped out his plan for reorganizing the profession and showed it to White.[16] It took the Commonwealth Fund less than a week to reject Sullivan's funding request for the Joint Committee. Its officers had turned for advice to White, Ruggles, and their close associate, Frankwood Williams.[17] Much abashed, Sullivan wrote White that "for reasons chiefly intuitive I feel that your active enthusiasm has not attached to this proposition," and he asked for reassurance. White's answer, delayed almost a month, was a study in circumlocution. Within two months Sullivan stepped down from the Joint Committee in favor of Franklin Ebaugh of the University of Colorado (a Meyer student). Funding from the National Committee for Mental Hygiene soon followed.[18] Ebaugh's eventual proposals made no mention of the social sciences; they did envision the establishment of the requirements for the specialty of psychiatry through an examining board under the American Psychiatric Association and the (AMA) National Board of Medical Examiners. In other words, Ebaugh's plan reflected psychiatry's ambition to become an accepted medical science.[19] The ensuing institutional integration of psychiatry with neurology in the new examining board and medical school curricula handcuffed psychiatry to the Jacksonian level theory. When that theory foundered in the 1950s, psychiatry was set adrift without a rudder.

Meanwhile, in mid-1931, Ebaugh's committee proposed a roundtable discussion on psychiatric education. Ebaugh sent a list of prospective participants to White for comment. Sullivan's name was absent, but White wrote that the list seemed complete.[20]

The 1934 creation of the American Board of Psychiatry and Neurology, under the joint auspices of the American Medical Association and the American Psychiatric Association, to control the qualifying of specialists, registered a further shift in power to the medical schools. But Sullivan had not given up. In late 1933 he organized the William Alanson White Foundation in Washington, D.C., as the engine for raising funds for a research and teaching institute to be named the Washington School of Psychiatry. He dreamed of a post-doctoral training center for social scientists and psychiatrists. Throughout 1935 he worked to enlist the gifted and innovative for his faculty — Edward Sapir, Harold Lasswell, Erich Fromm, Gordon Allport, Karen Horney, Frieda Fromm-Reichmann, and many others. The problem was money. White, exhausted and close to death, showed no interest.[21] Large grants never materialized. But the school, incorporated in 1936, became a center for intellectual ferment within the field of psychiatry.

As I have already noted, Sullivan's first (1924) publication was a slap in White's face. "The schizophrenic," he wrote there, "appreciates all too definitely the attitude of the physician. . . . Solipsism, excursions into phantasmagorical 'collective' and 'racial' unconsciousness . . . all these views bring to the patient much of the same destructive influences to which he was previously subjected in the world."[22] In short, White's approach was dehumanizing.

The next year, 1925, brought forth another Sullivan production (this time in White's own *Psychoanalytic Review*)—a shamelessly rough treatment of mental health liberalism's most cherished notion, community. The thesis is easily stated and profoundly important to all his later thought. It is simply that the differentiation into self versus objects comes during the oral phase—the lip-nipple disjunction—and incorporates into itself the fantastic project to dominate the environment. Language and culture reflect this project (by dividing the world into the self and not-self, for example). The child grows to adulthood with a subject-object consciousness structured by a fantastic and ego-centric language that he cannot escape. It is a consciousness contrary to reality and is readily collapsed and thus schizophrenia occurs. To avoid the collapse of our realities, we all develop security operations—operations that act to avoid a true consciousness of reality by building and reinforcing our self-esteem (thus reinforcing the Cartesian dualism). The schizophrenic is one whose security operations (powers of self-deception) are defective.[23] Sullivan had decided that the subject-object split is capable of being sustained only by a language burdened by fantastical elements. The schizophrenic's horror is that he lives in a collapsed world, but our horror is that our world is structured—perceptually and conceptually—by language and thought patterns that set one's self over against the world as subject against object, creating a constant opposition and an eternal exercise of dominance-submission.

Freud believed that the infant's world is a satisfying thing, defined by the mother's breast and love. Sullivan dissented. In "Oral Complex," he pictured a world terrifyingly defined by oxygen deprivation succeeded by hunger-induced anxieties. This was no life of infantile bliss or savage eroticism to which one might wish to escape in a schizophrenic break. The horror Sullivan imagined for the schizophrenic was matched only by the awfulness of the sort of world he found himself in—a world in which impersonal manipulations are disguised as love and devotion.

Friendship with anthropologist-linguist Edward Sapir, dating from the late 1920s, was extremely important to Sullivan. It meant an introduction into the myth-building properties of language and gave him an ally in his mission to demythologize schizophrenia. Sapir was already noted for his rebuttal of English evolutionary anthropology. With Franz Boas at Columbia University, he made mincemeat of the notion that there ever was a man whose mental processes were somehow more primitive (less abstract, more dream-like, more sexually dominated, and more stimulus-bound) than that of modern Western man. One of his most devastating pieces, now famous, was his contrast between the modern telephone switchboard girl and the Indian salmon fisherman, the one mechanized, routinized, and alienated by science and technology; the other living in organic union with his community and his natural environment. Nothing could more effectively puncture the higher-lower doctrine's mythology. Just as searching was his nominalistic insistence that the word "society" is an abstraction. There is no such thing; there is only the interaction between individuals at a given moment in time.[24]

James had long since convincingly placed the individual within the stream, thereby shutting him or her off from any world of enduring realities save by the ultimately spurious act of abstraction. Holt, and following him, White, had extracted themselves by proposing an emergent lawfulness and structure. How else explain what James was unable to explain to the satisfaction of his critics—how two people can know the same thing—unless there is a theory of emergent structure to provide a stable world? Sapir had a different answer. Two people structure the world in the same way because they speak the same language: "Language, as a structure, is on its inner face the mold of thought."[25] Sapir's outer world remained as unstructured and as unknowable as did Kant's. And, since all structure remains arbitrary, one language (no matter how primitive) gives a structure as legitimate as the next. Or, as illegitimate.

Shortly after he left Sheppard-Pratt in 1931 to take up private practice in New York, Sullivan notified White that he was working on a book. *Personal Psychopathology*, completed about 1932, was not published in Sullivan's lifetime. The reasons are obscure. Certainly White showed no enthusiasm—this may have been a possible factor. On the other hand, Sullivan often noted his inability to communicate in writing. He carried in his head the picture of his reader, a "bitterly paranoid . . . very brilliant thinker, and at the same time an extraordinary wrong-headed imbecile," who maliciously perverted Sullivan's meanings, yet could not comprehend the simplest of his ideas: "The result is, as I say, that I write almost nothing."[26] Sullivan, whose "interpersonal theory" of psychiatry leaned heavily on the idea of mental health through "consensual validation," was so impressed by the difficulties of communicating ("parataxic language") that he could not shake his feelings of isolation and of being locked into his own thoughts and perceptions. But consider the paradox he faced: "Consensual validation" makes for mental health — the reinforcement of a person's beliefs secures that person in his or her own reality — but the reigning consensual validation in America locks everyone into a spurious I-it relation with the world and with others that doubly isolates, first by creating an aggressive attitude of impersonal control toward the world, second by mystifying that attitude as love. Is it any wonder that some people — people we call schizophrenic — opt out?

Freud, beyond doubt a greater mind than Sullivan, had found a home in the old household, had refurbished it, and had made it habitable for yet one more generation. But Sullivan found himself cast out, a wanderer over new terrain. Freud, the speculative genius, dealt still with the familiar, the higher-lower doctrine and multiple personality theory, and so had an inner certainty of what he was about — he had consensual validation. Sullivan could have no such security. As he thought and wrote, his sense of isolation increased.

Sullivan leaned heavily on the notion of the conscious "I" and the unconscious "not-I," which Kempf had developed in *The Autonomous Functions and the Personality.* Yet *Personal Psychopathology* was a new departure. In it the "I" becomes the "good-me," quite as Kempf intended, but the "bad-me," the socially disapproved me, is not unconscious in Sullivan's statement; it is part of our everyday conscious baggage. In *Personal Psychopathology,* and in his 1940 "Conceptions of Modern Psychiatry," Sullivan described still a third sort of selfhood — a "not me" — to handle what Kempf had described as the unconscious.[27]

Sullivan's theory of multiple selves drew on the idea that one gains a sense of self from the way others (most importantly, one's mother) respond toward one. Certain behavior elicits friendly responses (the "good mother"), others elicit hostile responses (the "bad mother").

Thus each of us normally develops two basic self structures, the "good-me" and the "bad-me." But we will exclude from attention (thus from our "self-systems") such of our own behaviors that are too anxiety provoking—the "not-me" is born. Sullivan called this process "selective inattention," and substituted it for the Freudian unconscious. Gone, therefore was the unconscious as embodiment of the lower—the savage, the machine, the dream.

Sullivan felt that the "bad me" dominates the schizophrenic patient. In his case, the smile of appreciation, the friendly greeting, and the gesture of approval remain unattended to. This can happen when a child's mother is herself so full of anxiety that her attitudes toward her child are hopelessly ambiguous. And how could it be otherwise, given our culture in which love is disguised manipulation? The schizophrenic patient was never able to integrate a conception of his mother that he could count on. His "bad-me" developed as a counterpart to his threatening world, his ambiguous mother. Thus the schizophrenic retreats, even to the point where he denies reality itself to the world.[28]

But certainly the hostile, unpredictable world from which the patient retreats was anything but unreal to Sullivan. It was a world predicated upon the fantasy of domination—a fantasy built into the language and growing out of the oral complex. He became dissatisfied with the simple "good-me," "bad-me" division. He conceived of certain events (for example, prenatal conception of death, the immediate post-partum oxygen hunger, and so on) too devastating to be integrated with a self-system. Other events occurring after the self-system begins to develop may be too horrendous and anxiety-provoking for integration, lest the self-system crumble. Thus, the "not-me," the antithesis of a self-system. It can be the collapse of the self-system, indeed of one's whole world.[29]

Sullivan's "not-me" was not an evil me, it was a state of disintegration. It was not the Freudian unconscious, not Hall's savage, not Prince's somnambulist, and not White's racial past. Those had all been metaphorical ways of disguising the non-Cartesian perceptual orientation. In Sullivan's "not-me" that perceptual orientation comes into the open out from behind its disguises. In the "not-me" the individual becomes one with the whole world of the "not-self," the world of alien objects. One's self becomes an alien object. The "not-me" becomes conscious when the subject-object supporting cultural mythology is shattered for the individual. At the same time, the "not-me" is the product of that cultural mythology and the actions it supports. It is the product of being acted upon as an object by others from whom one has been misled to expect love.

While relating these kinds of observations not long before his death in 1948, Sullivan paused to comment to his audience on two myths. One was Mark Twain's *Mysterious Stranger*, the unremittingly gloomy statement of scientific naturalism. The story here, according to Sullivan, was about a good boy who kept asking his friend Satan to help people in trouble. Satan would comply, then the normal course of events would bring far more trouble to those he had helped. This was Sullivan's comment on the "evils of the transcendental power at the disposal of man"—that is, the ability to intervene into natural processes.[30] Scientific naturalism's appeal lies in order, but Twain's myth, by Sullivan's account, despairingly tells us that order is aimless and impersonal. The world that Sullivan believed he saw through the eyes of his patients was aimless chaos. The schizophrenic's dissolution, his objecthood, his "not-me," lurks within the impersonality of his mother's manipulations.

Sullivan related this tale without comment, but assuredly he was thinking of man's fantastic project to dominate. It is enough to consider the fact that he was speaking to an audience of dedicated psychotherapists, trained in the doctor-patient relation, professionals, whose higher-lower doctrine masked its reification of the I-it relation in the guise of therapeutic concern.

His second myth was that of Balaam and the ass. Sapir had recounted the biblical story and got him to think about it. Balaam, off on a mission for his town, began beating his ass when it balked on the road. The ass asked why. Had it not been a faithful servant? Balaam grew ashamed, the scales fell from his eyes, and he saw an angel blocking the way. Although unsettled by the notion of a talking animal, Sullivan thought it through, deciding, finally, that it was a tale of man's exalted consciousness leading him blindly along paths predetermined by cultural idealizations until a "deeper, older part of the personality" sees through the fallacy.[31] The promptings of the heart are better than the conceptualizations that ensnare the mind.

A note of hope had entered Sullivan's thinking, a note carried over from the Jelliffe-White creative racial mind, Putnam's creative child, and Prince's Sally. It had its sources in Meyer's attempts to go behind abstractions to the human individual and perhaps even in James's journey of the sick soul through its own private hell into a redeemed life. Sullivan's schizophrenic was one from whose eyes the scales had fallen; one who, though desperately ill, is set free to experience the deeper sort of human relation.

Sullivan was able to enter imaginatively into the schizophrenic patient's world. His natural sympathy was part of the story, as were Sapir's insights into language and Sullivan's consequent freedom from the higher-lower doctrine. He thus stood outside the professional's role vis-à-vis the patient, becoming aware of the profound ambiguity pervading our interpersonal relations. The child senses the manipulative techniques hidden within the mother's manifestations of loving concern and discovers its own objecthood, its "not-me." For her part, the mother is locked into her I-it relation by her culture and by the fact that her cultural mythology masks her impersonal manipulations. In discovering this, Sullivan knew he had unmasked the doctor-patient relation and its supporting mythology.

Sullivan's demythologizing mission profoundly influenced American psychiatry. He robbed psychiatry of its savage. His colleagues found a new home for the lower in the "oral incorporative" infant, but we shall see that metaphor as a mark of the higher-lower doctrine's declining state. More devastatingly, Sullivan replaced the emergent community with the vision of a society built upon culturally masked alienation. His successors would begin to wonder if what we call mental health does not, after all, consist in our ability to be at home with self-delusion. Above all, Sullivan sounded the message of the schizophrenic patient's essential humanity. It is a commentary on the state of psychiatric practice that his message was a destabilizing one. Belief in the schizophrenic's humanity had no place in the established doctor-patient relation, predicated as it was on the notion that it is the doctor's job to bring the schizophrenic back into humanity. Sullivan left his colleagues a legacy of self-doubt and hurried them along into the next phase of the dialectic of objectification.

In his 1914 essay "On Narcissism," Freud placed the psychotic beyond the pale of psychoanalytic therapy. The psychotic seemed unreachable. Bleuler and Jung had added their large authority to this conclusion. Yet several people trained in psychoanalysis or in Freudian theory made the attempt: Kempf and Sullivan in America, Melanie Klein and W. R. D. Fairbairn in England. Others were encouraged to found private hospitals devoted to psychoanalytically-oriented treatment of schizophrenic patients: Chestnut Lodge in Rockville, Maryland; the Forest Sanatorium, Des Plaines, Illinois; and to some extent, the Menninger Clinic, Topeka, Kansas. From the staffs of these and from some older centers in Baltimore, Boston, New York and Chicago, a subgroup of schizophrenia-oriented psychiatrists, decidedly nonorthodox in their Freudianism, emerged in the post-World War II period. Their theoretical departure from Freud grew largely from the work of Sullivan, Klein, and Fairbairn.

The schizophrenic they saw is rather an old friend of ours by now. Robert Knight of the Austen Riggs Foundation wrote that the "schizophrenic's defenses against primitive instinctual impulses, ancient memories, and archaic, infantile ways of dealing with the world have broken down, and the unconscious content has flooded into conscious awareness."[32] Norman Cameron, a Meyer student, based his approach on the proposition that "practically all of the symptoms of schizophrenia are results of the emergence of primary process material into secondary process thinking."[33] C. Peter Rosenbaum put it more graphically: "The moat is empty; the bridge is down; the sentinels fail to stand guard. The unconscious storms into consciousness, and the waking dreamer of Jung is to be seen." Silvano Arieti of Chestnut Lodge put it simply: "How can we tell a patient, 'Your life is a dream. Wake up'?"[34]

The schizophrenic as waking dream harkens back to turn-of-the-century theory, but now a new element is added: having swallowed the patient's consciousness, the dream was now seen as reaching out to swallow up the psychiatrist. We turn to this development.

Freud himself did spadework for the new departure in his "On Narcissism" and in various papers on transference and countertransference. In "On Narcissism" he concluded that the psychotic patient has regressed to infant narcissism, a stage described in *Three Essays on the Theory of Sexuality*[35] as oral and as solipsistically self-sufficient. Following up on that, Karl Abraham, of the inner circle, divided that infantile stage into "oral dependent" (sucking) and "oral incorporative" (biting), thus setting the scene for the Klein-Fairbairn advance.[36]

In 1941, W. R. D. Fairbairn, working with schizophrenic patients, announced a radical departure in libido theory: the so-called anal and phallic phases of psychosexual development are mere artifacts of earlier oral developments, and, therefore, the Freudian theory of the psychoses is wrong.[37] For those working with schizophrenics, it seemed a breakthrough. Fairbairn argued that as the gratifying breast advances and retreats, the infant learns to respond with love and hate toward the mothering object (that is, the mother). The infant learns both acceptance and rejection; the mother comes to be both the good object and the bad—the "good-bad mother." In the perception of any infant, the mother becomes two people. But, argued Fairbairn, the schizophrenic patient never gains the ego strength to reintegrate his object world. It remains split into the good and the bad.

Fairbairn tried to capture his sense of the schizophrenic patient's infantile helplessness with a small animal metaphor. "It is at once fascinating and pathetic to watch the patient, like a timid mouse, alternately creeping out of the shelter of his hole to peep at the world of outer objects and then beating a hasty retreat."[38] This sense of the schizophrenic's helplessness became widespread. It largely repeated Sullivan's perception of the individual whose world has collapsed. "Increase in unpleasure to the point of the ego's feeling overwhelmed," wrote Elvin Semrad, "is met by a body response of disintegration, terror, fear, panic and dread."[39] Donald Jackson of Stanford University wrote that "the patient is helpless and in need. The therapist could have the same feelings in relation to a . . . sick dog."[40]

But the small animal metaphor was less popular than the helpless infant. Louis Hill, psychiatrist-in-chief at the Sheppard-Pratt hospital, said, in his widely-read book of 1955, that the patient "finds sympathetic response in anyone who feels positively for newborn babies."[41] And if the patient is a helpless infant, locked (in fantasy) into infant-nipple symbiosis, then the psychiatrist must, in fantasy, be the mother's breast. The question is: In whose fantasy? We find some psychiatrists believing not only that they were mother's-breast surrogates, but that to play the role of breast was their job as therapists. And more, many of the psychiatrists did some fantasizing of their own. Speaking of therapist and schizophrenic patient, Semrad said, "The two have entered into each other's lives, serving as infantile objects."[42] Hill wrote that the patient's underlying drive "is to force the therapist to be a good breast, uncluttered by any disturbing attributes." He equated therapy with "parental love."[43] Leon Saul of the University of Pennsylvania Medical School told of a patient who was "like a hungry kitten given milk."[44] And Arieti wrote that with "the schizophrenic patient . . . I am not a peer. My role is nutritional and maternal."[45]

In their 1953 study, Carl Whitaker and Thomas Malone argued that analyst and patient must reestablish the mother-child relation.[46] How was this to be carried out in practice? Julius Steinfeld, Medical Director of Forest Sanatorium, related his practice of giving patients prolonged insulin or electroshock treatment forcing regression to a stage of infant-orality and thus allowing him to assume the role of good mother by supplying sweets. Then, wrote Steinfeld, the therapist finds in himself a "spontaneous, often fanatic, almost compulsive desire to help, to nurse, to support, to give."[47] John Rosen, noted for his "direct analysis," said that the therapist "must be the idealized mother who has now the responsibility of bringing the patient up all over again."[48] He told colleagues at the 1955 Sea Island Conference, "I say to the patient: 'Drink this good milk; my breast won't hurt your teeth the way your mother's did.' "[49]

The Sea Island conferees spoke of their feelings when "feeding" patients. Malcolm Hayward, University of Pennsylvania Medical School, said, "I have a wonderful feeling of euphoria." Thomas Malone, Atlanta Psychiatric Clinic, agreed: "I do afterwards." Carl Whitaker, of the same clinic, related how he would suck his own tongue as if he were the baby "sucking myself," during those times "when it is very clear that I am feeding the patient, and I feel as if I were both the mother and the patient at the same time." "That," said Malone, "is my feeling exactly." Whitaker described massaging the patient's foot as a "feeding experience," and John Warkentin of the Atlanta Psychiatric Clinic described his "warmth and happiness" when putting patients on his lap.[50]

Clearly these gentlemen were good mothers in fantasy as well as theory. Just as clearly, to them their adult patients really were infants.

But those were extreme expressions. Probably most therapists believed it wrong to carry the good-breast role that far.[51] It was thought, for one thing, that the practice might lock the patient into fantasy; for another thing, the fantasy included the therapist as "bad breast," and that might cause problems. But another aspect of this drawing back from the role of the mother was the patient's apparent fragility—what I will call the "fragility of the object."

The belief developed that the state of schizophrenia was the patient's last tenuous hold upon reality, that the least mistake might send the patient tumbling. Frieda Fromm-Reichmann, who, after fleeing Nazism in 1935, remained for twenty-two years at Chestnut Lodge to exert enormous influence, wrote: "The love which the sensitive schizophrenic feels as he first emerges and his cautious acceptance of the analyst's warmth of interest are really most delicate and tender things. . . . [The analyst] may easily freeze to death what has just begun to grow and so destroy any further possibility of therapy."[52] Here again the little mouse peeps from its hole. Hill wrote that "withdrawal and regression, impulsive outbursts, anything from catatonic stupor to catatonic excitement, may be the patient's only comment upon a broken appointment, a tactless remark, or the therapist's observed attention to another patient."[53] Donald Burnham, former Director of Research at Chestnut Lodge and editor of *Psychiatry*, noted that a "brief glance out of the window, a shift in his chair, or a deep breath by the doctor" might signal abandonment.[54] Burnham said the schizophrenic patient's desperate need for a stable relationship comes from a good-bad mother whose inconsistent personality blasts the child's hold on reality. When the psychiatrist plays the good mother he is tempting fate.

Psychiatrists saw the patient's labile perceptual processes as the problem: the most innocent gesture might signal rejection. But a look at the psychiatrist's perceptual processes argues that we put the shoe on the other foot: in the therapeutic situation the analyst's own hold upon the subject-object mode of perception became so tenuous that any sudden (unpredictable) behavior by the patient sent the analyst tumbling into the unknown—that is, into the non-Cartesian mode. This, of course, is the thesis I have been maintaining throughout. Sensitized by Sullivan, post-World War II psychiatrists were far more aware of their own subjective reactions. "The term 'archaic,'" wrote William Pious of the Menninger Clinic and of Yale, "includes not only the incomprehensibility and the quantity of idiosyncratic usage but also the degree of my sense of the 'uncanniness' of the behavior."[55] But, even more, the new psychiatric scene involved a shift in metaphors, from primitive dream on the Freudian model to the horror dream of the "not-me," now embodied in the term "oral incorporation."

The schizophrenic was still very much Jung's "waking dream," but he was far from being the analyzable dream of Freud.[56] He was the Storch-White loss of ego boundaries combined with the idea of infant narcissism—the fantasy of the good-bad breast. In his 1971 *Clinical Psychiatry*, an attempt to assess the latest work in the field, Hans Oppenheimer contrasted the Freudian (normal) dream with the mentality of schizophrenia in this way: "In a [normal] dream, unintelligibility may be both *intended* and *inflicted*. But can the same be said of . . . dementia praecox? Unlike the dream there is no latent element of which schizophrenic dementia is the distorted, let alone disguised, manifestation."[57] Freud's manifest dream content was a disguise of the latent dream (the infantile wishes). In Oppenheimer's schizophrenia the helpless infant stands undisguised in his unstructure. Theorists as diverse as Leopold Bellak, a graduate of an orthodox institute, and Norman Cameron, a Meyer student, agreed.[58] Freud's dream had a logical structure; if the new theorists were right, schizophrenic thought had none.

The psychiatrist's object was becoming fragile: at the slightest provocation, the patient ceased to be the helpless child—the peeping mouse—and dissolved into unstructure.

In terms reminiscent of Sullivan, Otto Allen Will of Chestnut Lodge described the patient's panic in the face of chaos. The therapist, said Will, tries to provide stability, but may "recoil from what he experiences as excessive demands on his energy, time, and emotions; he speaks of being devoured, manipulated, enveloped, and so on."[59] Writing of the youths at the New York Psychiatric Institute Children's Service, Margaret Mahler told of their insistence on being kissed and cuddled, and of their horror reaction at any show of affection. Mahler concluded that "their biting, kicking and squeezing the adult is the expression of their craving to incorporate, unite with, possess, devour and retain the 'beloved.' "[60] Steinfeld described the situation when the therapist becomes the bad breast and the patient becomes sadistic, consumed by "ravenous eating desires. . . . 'Eating up and destroying the mother's breast'."[61]

What I have called the fragility of the object involves the transformation of the small animal or helpless infant metaphor into its opposite.

The literature became flooded with horrendous images of the schizo-phrenic patient as cannibal.

Roy Grinker of the Michael Reese Hospital in Chicago wrote that when the ego structure breaks down, there will often be a revival of the cannibalistic oral patterns of infancy.[62] Burnham believed that the schizophrenic patient's reality has so disintegrated that he clings to any stable object, and "seeks absolutely to possess and to be pos-sessed by the object."[63] Other writers put (and felt) the matter more strongly. Richard Chessick wrote of "cannibalistic incorporation," and told of one patient's "enormously grasping, swallowing, and engulfing attitude and behavior. At worst it was a cannibalistic incorporative demeanor that she presented to me hour after hour."[64] Charles Savage, formerly of the Washington School of Psychiatry and the National Institute of Mental Health, spoke of the analyst's relation with the schizophrenic patient: "It is an intense oral-incorporative nature which exhausts the analyst and threatens him with loss of his identity."[65] At the South Island Conference, Whitaker mentioned a case of a patient fearing he would kill the therapist; perhaps the patient really thought he was going to eat him. Conferee Malone agreed, adding: "This is a recurrent theme in all our experiences."[66] Milton Wexler of the Menninger Clinic wrote of a patient who sought "to take me in, to incorporate me in the most literal way."[67] Oral incorporation was no theoretical abstraction for these psychiatrists. It was grounded in their emotions and perceptions. Entering one schiz-ophrenic woman's room was "like going inside her," to Burnham's staff.[68] Searles told of a colleague at Chestnut Lodge who experi-enced a corpulent female patient as a giant amoeba and quoted him as saying that during the long hours of analysis—hours of "terrible silences"—he had begun to fantasize: "I thought of the amoeba ingesting a particle of food—and ingesting me, actually."[69]

The "oral incorporation" metaphor translates into the therapist's fear of being incorporated. Savage's fear of loss of identity was not unique. "As each new patient-hour arrives," said Whitaker, "it's my own inner life that is at issue."[70] It was fine to play the role of the good breast, but disconcerting to discover oneself the object of fantasy. Beyond the fear of being devoured was the shock that one is but an abstraction for the patient. The I-it relation now turned back upon the doctor. Burnham recorded how anxiety had caused a patient to misperceive his analyst as someone else, whom the patient disliked. The analyst had not only shifted from good to bad object, thought Burnham, but to no real person at all.[71] Jurgen Ruesch was so struck by the schizophrenic's tendency to treat others as "nonidentifiable particles such as atoms or molecules," that he fantasized him as future man, "of homo sapiens as a species of frail body and oversized head," all mind and no heart.[72] Will spoke of the anxiety caused by being totally blocked out by the patient.[73]

The perception of being seen as other than themselves had a profound effect. Savage and Mabel Cohen of Chestnut Lodge believed they were obliged to play the abstraction good-bad mother and registered their anxiety.[74] Searles at times fantasized himself as a dehumanized monster in the eyes of his patients and, to his own consternation, reacted by feeling and acting monstrously towards them.[75] He believed he was becoming his patients' creation.

These kinds of anxieties made the psychiatrists sense an enormous power in the schizophrenic patient. On the one hand, even though the patient was felt to be abstracting and fantasizing and not seeing the psychiatrist as he really was, the patient was often credited with the power of seeing through the analyst's defenses and disguises to the hypocrite behind them. Savage wrote of a patient who perceptively told his analyst to try and overcome her homosexual tendencies. He credited the patient with a "sensitivity and perceptivity" gained from surviving in a hostile environment.[76] Fromm-Reichmann counseled total honesty with the patient, trained by experience to see through social rationalizations. The patient holds a mirror up to society and to the therapist.[77] Commenting on that, David Wright said that "inevitably, and with the most careful selection, the schizophrenic can pick out, and will pick out, the therapist's specific vulnerable points."[78]

This unmasking operation was believed to lay bare the psychiatrist's hitherto unconscious thoughts and wishes. Eugene Brody observed that "one of the most frequently mentioned features of the schizophrenic is his apparent sensitivity to unverbalized and sometimes only partially conscious feelings in the therapist."[79] Hill wrote that while the patient is unconscious of our reality, he "is conscious of that which is deeply unconscious in the doctor." How could this be? The psychiatrists felt that their patients beheld them only as abstractions. They agreed with Hill that the patient, "as Jung once put it . . . is in a waking dream."[80] How did these perceptions square with the feeling that the patient could see beyond his dream, beyond his abstracting, and deep into the psychiatrists' hidden recesses? The answer lies not in logic but in the dialectic. The psychiatrists perceived a raw unconsciousness rising to envelop them; a horror dream dragging them into itself. The patient's primitive unconscious seemed to call forth their own primitivity, their own unconsciousnesses. The metaphor, "oral incorporation," was closely related to the therapist's sense of being drawn into his own unconscious, his own dream. As Hill put it, the patient attempts to split the therapist in two; the therapist responds by splitting into a rational observer and a regressed, childish, fantasizing, and dominating person.[81]

One becomes an observer, watching oneself in helpless horror and astonishment. One feels oneself come under the control of impulses and compulsions. One calls this the rise of the lower, the savage, or the unconscious, within oneself. The schizophrenic is one who has this power over the therapist. Savage wrote that the therapist experiences "the patient's intense anxieties, fears, rages, lusts, and conflicts as his own."[82] Chessick reiterated the theme throughout his book, *How Psychotherapy Heals* (1969): the patient's "preoedipal longings" stir up in the therapist his own "deeply repressed longings"; direct confrontation with the patient's "intense cannibalistic incorporation fantasies" forces the therapist to defend against his own "primitive drives — which are invariably stirred up and resonate to the strivings of the patient."[83] Not only did the therapist feel himself drawn into the unconscious, he was hard put to distinguish between his own and that of the patient — the two were shared, they were found to resonate, the patient's unconscious was felt as his own. When describing the illness of the patient, this same phenomenon was inevitably called "loss of ego boundaries."

This, then, was the essence of the feeling for which the new metaphor "oral incorporation" stood: the sense of loss of one's own ego boundaries or selfhood, of being an abstraction without existence outside the patient's fantasy; the sense of being reduced to an object in the eyes of the other ("We are all too familiar with the 'schizophrenic stare.' Imagine the great tendency to resist being incorporated all day long by patients!"[84]); the sense of being lost in subjectivity ("By the end of the hour I felt as though I had been tied up within a package and sent tumbling over and over into a void."[85]).

The definition of a schizophrenic: someone who throws the observer into the non-Cartesian perceptual orientation. The definition of psychiatry: a defense against the non-Cartesian perceptual orientation.

The most elaborate and intense description of the process is found in the work of Harold Searles of Chestnut Lodge, who Austen Riggs Foundation director Robert Knight called "probably the most widely read and respected authority in the world on the psychotherapy of chronic schizophrenics."[86] As already mentioned, Searles found himself dehumanizing his patients. He described a female patient — short, heavy-set, powerful — and spoke of her most frightening "animal rage," saying that she seemed to have at least one foot in "the realm of savage beasts" during her "nonhuman periods." He described a particularly offensive male who spent much of the treatment hour belching, grunting, and passing flatus: "As those months wore on I found — initially, to my great dismay — that I could not help reacting to him as being more an offensive animal than a human being."[87]

This tendency to dehumanize led Searles to decide that the id or nonhuman aspect of the patient was forcing him, the analyst, to regress to the patient's nonhuman level. Searles analyzed the situation thus: The patient first depreciates outer reality (the therapist) to the point where it ceases to exist for him, then he tries to incorporate it. Soon both patient and analyst attempt to incorporate their own personalities within that of the other. And, finally, "there appeared many indications that the 'personality' of the other, within which each of us had been keeping his functioning personality incorporated, was actually in large part a fantasy personality formed of his own repressed and projected feelings."[88] In this involuted process of the psychiatrist's perceptual response, which suggests a hall of mirrors, there is no core personality or self to be found — in neither patient nor doctor.

We see the dialectic of objectification at work as we watch the helpless infant rise in rage and as the doctor feels the boundaries between himself and the outside world crumble, that is, as he finds himself being incorporated and swallowed-up. The dialectic is consumated in the psychiatrist's loss of ego boundaries. He has been thrown into the non-Cartesian dualism.

We work from a basic assumption: When perceived structure is threatened by the unpredictable, one works to reconstitute structure. One aspect is the assigning of the unpredictable to some residual category (for example, schizophrenia, the unconscious, the id), thereby leaving the remaining area of structure intact but diminished. The more we impose structure upon another person, the more his behavior will appear as unpredictable, and the residual category will grow. Pressure toward perceptual control acts to enlarge what we perceive as his irrationality.

Culture functions to maintain predictable behavior. Every culture, one supposes, must have its residual category—"the irrational."[89] Guardians of that category are assigned to keep it under control. In America the modern (official) guardians became the psychiatrists, and their advanced skirmish line was made of the men and women specializing in schizophrenia.

The metaphors psychiatry developed to handle the residual category worked only so long as they remained unrecognized as metaphor. Anthropology's rejection of evolutionary ethnology, with its savage, was a blow. In Sullivan's "not-me" the metaphors were shed entirely. The skirmish line faltered and retreated, reforming around the metaphor "oral incorporation." But it exposed as much as it hid in that it expressed the residue's relentless expansion at the expense of remaining perceptual structure.

Psychiatrists began to feel themselves demolished—"incorporated." When one can no longer anticipate the other person's behavior, one can no longer anticipate one's own. One finds one's own reactions becoming uncontrolled and unanticipated, and assigns those reactions to the "unconscious"—this time one's own. So the psychiatrists imagined that their patients had gained control over their own primitive wishes.

To break this cycle, Prince and his generation worked out the psychiatric edition of the doctor-patient relation and gave it definition with an ideology—mental health liberalism. That relation, paradigmatic for the new middle-class professional, defined a stable area of selfhood for both doctor and patient. The professional-client relations represented by the doctor and the patient was the twentieth-century replacement for tradition, custom, and inherited beliefs as the instrument for maintaining perceptual control. Relations guided by custom and inner controls were replaced with techniques of manipulation. The manipulative aspect of the new relations was kept secret from both parties so long as the metaphors remained persuasive.

It is perceived structure that selects from the infinity of experiencings, giving the selected ones a unity that we call an "object," and the impression that the object is "out there." Thus we may justly call the defining-out of a residual category part of the process of objectification.

But what of the residual category? Is it subject or object? My "unconscious" is not part of my subjectivity, nor is it part of the object world; it hangs in a never-never land between in here and out there. My anticipated actions are considered subjective ideas — they belong to me. But my unanticipated responses seem alien; they "just happen." They seem not-me. On the fringes of the subject-object world hovers the non-Cartesian world of the residue. When another person treats me as an object, my responses are likely to be of the unanticipated variety; I then become an object to myself through those alien responses. In this way, the patient becomes object to himself. The residual category — the patient's "unconscious" — grows in the eyes of the doctor. Desperately, in order to remain doctor, he presses forward with his objectification, and the patient becomes less and less able to respond as required. This is what Sullivan understood in his theory of the "not-me." But the profession could not listen to him and remain a profession. It opted instead for the new metaphor — "oral incorporation" — which perfectly described the doctor's deteriorating situation.

Had psychiatry kept hands off schizophrenia (as Freud counseled), the doctor-patient relation might have remained stable in the form given it by Prince and his generation. Yet without a solution to the problem of schizophrenia, psychiatry could not hold up its head as a science, nor as a therapy for mental illness. And this entailed the renewal of the dialectic.

At the heart of psychiatric theory, as well as of its ideology, mental health liberalism, lay the higher-lower doctrine. By watching its progress, we see how the dialectic got played out in the history of ideas. Prior to the idea of community preached by G. Stanley Hall, the doctrine simply envisioned a savage within — a lower being in whom reflective consciousness was absent. This was the lower level of Hughlings Jackson and the unconscious of Freud. However, in the typically American version of the doctrine as presented by Hall, the reflective consciousness was to be gained by shucking off isolating individualism and entering into community. This community, the new higher, was the alienated and reified selfhood of the doctor-patient relation writ large. Thus emerged mental health liberalism: the attainment of selfhood through action, for community controlled action lies in the domain of the object world and takes one out of the domain that is neither subject nor object, the domain of the residue.

Mental health liberalism depended for its power on metaphors. The savage fell by the wayside, partly because of advances in anthropology, partly because of the Sally theme in American psychiatry (the appeal of the free and spontaneous individual), submerged in Prince, growing in Putnam and Jelliffe, and dominant in Sullivan. But the events of the 1950s did not cause the demise of mental health liberalism, just its transformation. Its new form was presaged in the philosophy of Holt and the structuralism of White. It was no longer possible to blithely contrast community with savagery. A new language was needed.

7

PSYCHOSURGERY: SCIENCE CONFRONTS THE BIZARRE

The Real Miss Beauchamp was possible only when Sally was "killed." But, after World War II, faith in the possibility of dealing with her through psychotherapy was declining. Other methods were sought, and psychosurgery was one answer.

One of the most used descriptive terms for schizophrenia was the word "bizarre." Bleuler used the word over thirty times in his classic. The schizophrenic's ideas, he said, seem "bizarre" and "utterly unpredictable," they are "as strange as the birds which he feeds."[1] C. Macfie Campbell of the Harvard Medical School, wrote that "their emotional life, their motivation, their outlook on the world have a certain bizarre and unintelligible quality."[2] In 1947, J. M. Nielsen and George Thompson, speaking of incongruity between emotion and ideas in the schizophrenic, wrote that this "symptom may present itself in a most bizarre manifestation."[3] The term "bizarre" was given official sanction as a symptom in the American Psychiatric Association's 1968 definition of schizophrenia: "Behavior may be withdrawn, regressive and bizarre."[4]

Psychiatrists also liked "eerie," "strange," and "odd." A. A. Brill wrote in 1908 of "their strange utterances and peculiar behavior."[5] Oswald Boltz, of the Manhattan State Hospital, spoke of his schizophrenic patients as standing "before us like living question marks."[6] Karl Jaspers wrote that "All these personalities have something baffling about them . . . there is something queer, cold, inaccessible, rigid and petrified there."[7] And Adolf Meyer spoke of his schizophrenic patients' "oddity," "incongruity," and "unnaturalness."[8] One of Meyer's close colleagues, Phyllis Greenacre, wrote in 1918 that observing a schizophrenic is like "looking at a mutilated picture."[9] Greenacre's metaphor seems apt, but mutilated picture of whom?

156

Almost without exception, descriptions of the schizophrenic reflected feelings of coldness, reserve, and alienation. William Alanson White, for instance, said that the schizophrenic is characterized by his "Egyptian attitude, because we see the same attitude in the figures of Egyptian sculpture,"[10] an observation remindful of James's experience with the epileptic. The figure of speech suggests not only the exotic, but the alien. Another White statement suggests a blurring between the patient's emotions and White's own: "The fact [is] that the productions of the praecox strike us as being quite alien to us. We are not able to feel ourselves into the position which the praecox patient occupies."[11] To Boltz schizophrenics were "hypersensitive and cold at the same time," and, he added, to the "casual observer they seem to hold a pane of glass before them, so far and no further."[12] Jaspers wrote from Germany that "when faced with such people we feel a gulf which defies description."[13] A more recent authority, C. Peter Rosenbaum, after calling schizophrenics "aloof" people who make you feel their "contempt," made this instructive comment: "It is a frequent observation that the sudden appearance of anxiety in the interviewer, without his easily being able to find a reasonable explanation for its appearance, may be the first clue that he is dealing with a schizophrenic. This feeling is akin to the feelings of eeriness, awe, and dread that Sullivan ascribes to the 'Not-me'."[14] This was close to saying that the symptoms of schizophrenia lie in the subjective states of the psychiatrist himself.

This way of testing the patient was not new. Back in 1918 E. E. Southard of Boston's State Psychiatric Hospital made the patient's failure to pass the "empathy test" his quick, offhand, way of identifying a schizophrenic.[15] Southard's "empathy test," or "empathic index," speaks to psychiatry's approach down through the years. Nielsen and Thompson wrote that "there is a distinct feeling of strangeness one experiences in contact with the schizophrenic patient. . . . There is no empathy."[16] It became official when the American Psychiatric Association's *Diagnostic and Statistical Manual* stated that the schizophrenic's mood changes include the "loss of empathy with others."[17]

The awe, the dread, and the sense of the eerie that the psychiatrist felt were intimately related to his perception of the patient as unpredictable, unrelated, and distant. There is every reason to suspect that patients were often labeled schizophrenic because those feelings occurred in the psychiatrist.

In the 1920s and 1930s, despite minority dissent, it was generally concluded that schizophrenics are incapable of transfering their unconscious wishes onto the therapist and therefore incapable of analysis. Being the unconscious made conscious they could not acquire insight. In Gray's terms, they had lost the "conscious ego"—they were the truly insane. Such was Bleuler's, Freud's, and Jung's conclusion. "After spending an hour with a neurotic talking about his illness," wrote Bleuler, "some sort of personal relationship has been established, be it friendly or hostile. . . . Usually, however, it is impossible to establish any closer contact with schizophrenics (Jung)."[18] And Jung said: "Anyone who has penetrated the mind of an hysteric by analysis knows that he has gained moral power over the patient. . . . In dementia praecox, on the other hand, everything remains as before even after very thorough analysis. . . . They are and remain . . . uninfluenceable."[19] At St. Elizabeth's, White agreed with the majority, the archaic world of the schizophrenic patient was simply inaccessible to the analyst.[20]

The situation had not changed much by the 1950s:

> As Eileen's symptoms progressed, the therapies became correspondingly more drastic. A hysterectomy [!] was strongly recommended but never performed. She was given repeated courses of electroshock and insulin coma therapy, both separately and in combination. Hormonal treatments of various types were attempted. A lobotomy was strongly recommended, but not done. Psychotherapy was never attempted, not once.[21]

When faith was lost in analytic methods, other means were tried: drugs, shock, and psychosurgery. A look at the psychosurgery movement and its theoretical basis will suggest the lengths to which perceptual control was pursued. For some, dehumanization was not allowed to stand in the way of the fight against ambiguity.

Of the various surgical approaches, lobotomy and leukotomy were the most massive: lobotomy severed the connections between frontal lobes and much of the rest of the brain, leukotomy extirpated the lobes. These operations had their heyday in the 1940s before more precise surgical methods were substituted. Estimates of lobotomy operations generally run to 20,000. Lobotomy's leading popularizers and practitioners in America were Walter Freeman and James Watts (both of St. Elizabeth's), who worked together. They cut in the name of Hughlings Jackson (whom they often cited) and the higher-lower doctrine.[22]

The story of prefrontal lobotomy goes back in part to Harvard physiologist Walter Cannon's long fight against the James-Lange theory of emotion and James's elimination of mental events from the causal chain in behavior. James's 1884 "What is an Emotion?" stated that when confronted by a stimulus (for example, a bear), one responds (for example, runs), then one's emotion is largely the afferent sensations flowing into the brain from the responding organs. Jacksonians were soon working to refute the theory. In 1904 Sherrington and Woodworth in England found that decerebrated cats, when stimulated, showed rage responses.[23] This rage was "pseudoaffective," they reasoned, because without the cortex there could be no consciousness and hence no subjective feeling of emotion. Again in England, Head and Holmes attempted to pinpoint the center for emotions (pleasure and pain) in the thalamus, a portion of the brain tucked up inside the cerebral hemispheres and through which most sensations must pass before arriving at the various sensory areas of the cortex.[24]

Early in the 1920s Cannon concluded that the thalamus is indeed the seat of the emotions. He was followed by his Harvard student Philip Bard, who cut away ("ablated") most of the thalamus, leaving only the hypothalamus, and still found the rage response.[25] Cannon's thalamus (or, Bard's hypothalamus) was assumed to be a Jacksonian lower integrative level. Following Sherrington, Cannon assumed that without a cortex emotion cannot be subjectively experienced, and hence the rage emotion expressed was "sham": ergo, bodily expression and subjective experience are two different things. In the Jacksonian context, wherein consciousness begins at a high level, the Sherrington-Cannon conclusion made sense. Furthermore, Cannon had his students inject adrenin, with resulting "dilation of the bronchioles, constriction of blood vessels, liberation of sugar from the liver, stoppage of gastro-intestinal" and other visceral functions wherein James had partly located emotion. The students said they were unable to distinguish any specific emotions with those processes and Cannon concluded that there must be a subjective aspect to emotion—that is, its specificity—not accounted for by James.[26] He decided that James had left out the "glow and color to otherwise simply cognitive states."[27]

Yet, as Donald Hebb has pointed out, Cannon's critique of James was simply beside the point, an "extraordinary *non sequitur.*" James argued only against mental events intervening in the causal chain between stimulus and response—emotion is an afferent from the body to the brain, not an efferent signal to the body.[28] Locating an integrative function in the thalamus did nothing to argue for such an intervention. Why, then, all the fuss? Was Cannon really so ignorant of James? Hardly; not when he counted as "guide, philosopher, friend," the leading James interpreter, Ralph Barton Perry.[29]

We must look in another direction for the source and thrust of Cannon's assault. James left no room for a lower or a savage and no hidden explanation for the unexpected and bizarre. But this is just what the thalamus was for Cannon. James's theory, he wrote, "pays little or no attention to the always present and sometimes overwhelming *impulsive* aspect of the [emotional] experience. The localization of the reaction patterns for emotional expression in the thalamus . . . accounts . . . for the impulsive side . . . the sense of being seized, possessed, of being controlled by an outside force and made to act without weighing of the consequences."[30] We need to distinguish between the "archaic portion" of the nervous system and its newer parts. The archaic or primitive part accounts for "the mystery and surprise of an emotional outburst."[31]

Like Freud, Cannon was searching for the source of the compulsive self. Freud's answer was the unconscious, Cannon's the thalamus and the sympathetic nervous system it serves. For Cannon, the perceptual embodiment of compulsion was the "sham rage" of his cats. The sense of oneself as a detached and threatening usurper whom one watches in helpless anguish got itself lodged in a piece of anatomy.

Cannon's theory became controlling for American brain physiology and neurology. Bard shifted the seat of emotion slightly to the hypothalamus, and others, notably James Papez and Paul MacLean, shifted it again to an interaction between the hypothalamus and a group of parts they began to call the "visceral brain."

The Cannon-trained Stanley Cobb, of the Harvard Medical School, became a standard-bearer for the doctrine.[32] Cobb's 1949 Salmon Lectures show us how controlling the Jacksonian scheme remained. It had been found that the "sham rage" reaction was not similarly to be found in decorticated primates, nor, as it might be supposed, in man. Cobb duly noted the fact and laid it aside, putting the higher-lower doctrine (in somewhat new guise) as accepted theory. The cortex is divided into three levels, he said: the new cortex ("neocortex"), the middle cortex ("mesacortex"), and the old cortex ("archicortex"). The old cortex, or "visceral brain," "seems to have much to do with emotion and emotional expression.... It seems to set the emotional background on which man functions intellectually." Cobb suggested a comparison between the visceral brain and the Freudian id.[33]

In 1928, at the Peter Bent Brigham Hospital across the street from where Bard was producing "sham rage" in Cannon's laboratory, John Fulton watched an operation in which a few drops of Zenker's solution accidentally fell into the hypothalamic region. On recovery, the patient intermittently exhibited "sham rage" symptoms, which started Fulton to experiment in an effort to reproduce and to eliminate that sort of behavior. In 1935, he read a paper at the London International Neurological Congress on frontal lobectomies he and Carlyle Jacobsen were performing on chimpanzees, claiming to have transformed them into friendly creatures.[34] Egas Moniz took this information back to Lisbon, and, with a neurosurgeon, did lobotomies on twenty human patients, claiming success. The movement spread fast, with Freeman and Watts taking the lead in America. Looking back in 1951, Fulton, by then Sterling Professor of Physiology at Yale, provided (again) the theoretical basis for the movement he helped found by opening with a homage to Hughlings Jackson, "one of the ablest clinical observers in the annals of neurology," whose "influence upon neurological thought was probably greater than that of any other Englishman."[35]

On turning to the actual lobotomists, we find two major groups: the Freeman-Watts duo in Washington, D.C., operating out of the Jelliffe-White tradition, with heavy emphasis on Cannon; and a Harvard University group (Greenblatt, Solomon, and associates), influenced by a Stanley Cobb critique of the Freeman-Watts lack of theoretical rigor. Both groups were tightly bound by the Jacksonian paradigm, and both made it clear that the socially malleable and reduced human being was preferable to the bizarre, involuted, and unpredictable schizophrenic.

From its founding in 1934 until 1946, Walter Freeman was Secretary of the American Board of Psychiatry and Neurology. There he presided over the certification of all new neurologists and psychiatrists. He was a man of power. His Jacksonian bias seeped through his writings.[36] He pictured the frontal lobes as the highest level and the seat of self-consciousness. In an analysis that takes one back to the self-control trap, he reasoned that schizophrenia occurs in individuals preoccupied with abstract speculations, with resulting loss of energy, preoccupation with the self, and final surrender of mind to that lower level, the thalamus, "the organ par excellence of affective experience."[37]

For Freeman and Watts, all schizophrenics live in dreamy abstraction, are subject to hallucinations, and ruled by a runaway thalamus. Hallucinations and compulsive ideas were to be literally cut away by severing the thalamus's neural projections to the frontal lobes. The two men did not expect lobotomy to restore the patient to the levels of creative thought and personal initiative; on the contrary, by severing connections with the highest center, as they thought, they were eliminating those things in the elimination of subjective feeling. This, of course, was the Cannon-Bard line of reasoning. Relieved of subjectivity, the patients were free to return to the real world. Or, so thought Freeman and Watts.[38]

Getting clients to undergo treatment involved the two doctors in small intrigues, such as luring an unsuspecting individual into a hotel room where electroshock apparatus lay in wait. A series of shocks quieted the individual nicely, preparing him for the larger one to come. The results in terms of docility seemed gratifying. A three-hundred-pound "negress" struck terror in the breasts of her St. Elizabeth attendants. After lobotomy "we could playfully grab Ortha by the throat, twist her arm, tickle her in the ribs and slap her behind without eliciting anything more than a wide grin or hoarse chuckle." Even more to the point: "perhaps the greatest change . . . lies in their facial expression. . . . Lines of fatigue and exhaustion . . . make way for pleasant smiling countenances, a little vapid at times."[39]

Cloaked as he was in Jacksonian armor, Freeman was impervious to barbs, such as those he received from Harry Stack Sullivan.[40] When Cobb (1944) commented on their conceptual looseness, suggesting that vague phrases about "self-consciousness" and "imagination" be replaced with the idea of frontal lobe-thalamic reverberating circuits, Freeman and Watts gladly obliged: "One can," they wrote, "almost visualize the neural circuits in the frontal lobes vibrant with

activity. . . . The active circuits incorporate others into the new complex that grows and grows in depth and grandeur until something
snaps in the head."[41] How "until something snaps in the head" is an
advance in conceptual rigor was not explained. Apparently Freeman
and Watts had all the theoretical refinement they needed in those
smiling, vapid faces.

Cobb's sowing, however, found more fertile ground. The Greenblatt-
Solomon study done at the Boston Psychopathic Hospital, and reported
in 1953, used Cobb's "long-circuiting" idea. Greenblatt and Solomon
argued that the "long-circuiting" neural structures in the frontal lobes
get overcharged with excitation when instinctual drives are repressed.
Circuit overactivity blocks appropriate adaptation to the external world.
The result, they argued, is a progressive disorganization of the personality. The frontal lobe circuits, they felt, are responsible for the
repression of the id (which they seem to have equated with the
sympathetic nervous system in the manner of Kempf and Cannon) by
displacing energies onto themselves. Severing the links between those
lobes and the id would end repression and release energies for
adapting to reality.[42]

Greenblatt and Solomon were happy with their results and rec-
ommended the continued use of psychosurgery in less massive forms
than lobotomy. Wherein lay their success? According to their study,
most intellectual functions remained the same after the operation, but
thought processes became less bizarre and more coherent.[43] Moreover, marked hostility dropped from 68 percent to 18 percent of
those patients processed. "Finally, good impulse control, essentially
absence of unpredictable explosive outbursts, was present in 10 per
cent of cases before operation and 60 per cent of cases after operation."[44] Predictability and pleasantness—that constituted the success.
The fact that they found the postoperation patient to be mechanistically
sunk into the stimulus-response chain ("stimulus bound") did nothing
to dampen their enthusiasm. As they said: "Changes in social behavior for the average patient following operation indicate an enormous
improvement in social adaptation."[45]

Lobotomy (psychosurgery) was an expression of declining faith in
psychotherapy, but it was not so very different in its motivating premises. Many neurosurgeons were skeptical about its effectiveness. The
journals, while sometimes critical of its lack of clear-cut success,

generally took a wait-and-see attitude. Of the hundreds of articles devoted to discussing lobotomy, only a tiny minority pronounced against it outright, and then never on the basis of its inhumanity. In those years, the higher-lower doctrine was still quite strong, and in its terms, the operation made sense. The somewhat more sophisticated reverberating circuit theory—the view advanced by Cobb, Penfield, Kubie, and others—was not seen as an alternative to the Cannon-Bard approach. It dampened enthusiasm for massive intervention as such, but in 1950 a much more important event was about to happen—the higher-lower doctrine was about to fall.

It is clear that had James been taken seriously by American neurologists, lobotomies would never have been performed. They resulted from the dominance of Jacksonian level theory, the higher-lower doctrine, and the metaphors. In the early 1950s, the practice of radical psychosurgery (outside the area of epilepsy) sharply diminished, a fact that can be partly explained by a further turn of the wheel of neurophysiological theory. I have spoken somewhat of the foothold Jacksonian theory got in American physiology in the work of Cannon and his students, but more needs to be said of the associated mythology.

Stanley Cobb was a weathervane for all the latest theories. We can take his statements as representing the mainstream of his profession. By the 1940s, when Cobb's reputation was at its height, neurologists in America viewed the human brain as a sort of laminated affair, composed of three phylogenetic layers. At the bottom of the evolutionary scale, said Cobb, stands the "archipallium," composed of parts like the thalamus, hypothalamus, amygdala and epithalamus. This "old brain," tucked away underneath the cortex, was also called the rhinencephalon (smell brain), and/or the "visceral brain." In joining this group of suborgans into a system, Cobb was following James Papez and Paul MacLean. Next in line, thought Cobb, came the "mesapallium," which was of little importance to theory. Finally, we reach the "neopallium," the cortical mantle: "The neopallium thus truly becomes a cloak that covers the old brain almost completely."[46] The same scheme was still in use in the 1970s.

Cobb was putting things in proper perspective when he cited Papez and MacLean as his authorities. These were leading contemporary theorists on the structure of the brain. But, somewhat unexpectedly,

Cobb reached back in time to a turn-of-the century English morphologist-turned-anthropologist, G. Elliot Smith, as an authority. It was Smith who, in 1901, first coined the word "neopallium" and gave the twentieth century its phylogenetically-defined layered brain. Smith's layers were designed to accommodate and elaborate upon Hughlings Jackson's level theory. Since there was neither morphological nor clinical evidence to support his conclusions, Smith turned to the shrew.

It was clear to Smith that the "archipallium" in man is the same brain that occupies the skull of the ground shrew. This creature is pretty much dependent upon its nose and hardly at all upon its eyes (ears are not mentioned). Because he is dependent on his nose, his brain can be thought of as a "smell brain." When the shrew began its gradual evolution towards human form by climbing trees—that is, became a tree shrew—things had to change, the "neopallium," or new brain, started to evolve. "The high specialization of the sense of sight," Smith wrote, "awakened in the creature the curiosity to examine the objects around it with closer minuteness and supplied guidance to the hands in executing more precise and more skilled movements."[47]

Such was the sway of Jacksonian level theory that Smith's speculations were taken at face value. Of primary importance for Smith's impact in America was the fact that University of Chicago neurologist C. Judson Herrick made Smith's layered brain and associated arguments central to his own theory. In Herrick's influential book, *Brains of Rats and Men* (1920), Smith's layered brain blossomed forth in full neurophysiological dress. Herrick argued that in higher animal forms the cortex developed as the integrative level for the exteriorceptors (sight, hearing, touch), taking over that function from the thalamus of lower animals. The thalamus then joined the hypothalamus (forming the "diencephalon") as the seat of the emotions. Because at that time Karl Lashley at Johns Hopkins was raising suspicion toward the idea that the frontal lobes are the center for abstracting and generalizing, Herrick was forced to visualize a new idea of their function. He argued for a circuit between the frontal lobes and the thalamus, giving the frontal lobes the job of integrating emotion (from the thalamus) into the frontal (motor) field of the cerebral cortex.[48] Herrick had been brought to conclusions not unlike those of Cannon:

We have "old brain" and "new brain." Our conscious experience is also of two grades, the old mind that goes with the old brain and the new mind that goes with the new brain. The old mind is chiefly emotional and impulsive with flashes of intelligent understanding; this is the thalamic mind which we probably share with the lower animals. The new mind, or cortical mind, includes all the higher intellectual powers, our refined sentiments, and our voluntary control of conduct.[49]

Thus the villain of the plot, the source of our raw emotion and uncontrollable impulses, turns out to be the ground shrew, who somehow has made its nest in our brains.

When, in the 1940s, Stanley Cobb surveyed the state of neurophysiological theory, he placed his authoritative stamp of approval on the synthesis Herrick had produced. The Elliot Smith phylogenetic brain layers were to be allowed to stand. But for the latest and best theoretical work on emotion he turned to Papez and MacLean.

By 1937, the waters of emotion theory had become quite muddied. Cannon had argued for the thalamus as the seat of emotion, but Bard discovered the same "pseudo-affective," or, "sham" rage response after ablating the thalamus in cats. Meanwhile, few if any anatomical connections could be found to associate the hypothalamus with the "neopallium," a true hardship. Later, in 1939, in a now classic experiment on monkeys, H. Klüver and P. C. Bucy seemed to locate a seat for rage in the temporal lobes (that is, perhaps the amygdala).[50] At this crucial moment—1937—James Papez stepped into the breach to give the thalamic theory (and thus the higher-lower doctrine) a new lease on life based on the idea of cortical circuits.

Again it was Herrick who provided a point of departure for myth-saving theory. In 1933, Herrick had liberated the "archipallium" from its purely olfactory function by placing it in the "limbic system" and suggesting for the whole a function of non-specific activation.[51] Papez suggested that the old "smell brain" be recast as the seat of the emotions in the form of a circuit operating in the following fashion: "It is proposed that the hypothalamus, the anterior thalamic connections, the gyrus cinguli, the hippocampus and their interconnections constitute a harmonious mechanism which may elaborate the functions of central emotion, as well as participate in emotional expression."[52]

The whole complex circuit was to be seen as corresponding to the "old brain" residing beneath the neocortex.

Papez's services to the higher-lower doctrine went beyond bringing specific anatomical structures into a circuit configuration. By 1937, the idea of "seats," or "centers," was distinctly frayed at the edges. Every time a center was designated, it faded under closer inspection. Cannon's thalamus gave way to Bard's hypothalamus, which in turn was the victim of the Klüver-Bucy experiments. So, though Papez did fall back on center theory in suggesting that the "seat of consciousness" might be found in the gyrus cingulum, he did much better than that for emotion. Jackson, not liking the idea of centers, had used the notion of integrative levels. Cannon had something like that in mind when he described the function of the thalamus as refining emotion into subjective feeling, but he wanted nevertheless to pinpoint the savage in a definite center. Papez introduced the word "elaborate." His mechanism "elaborates" emotion, he said. The word soon became ubiquitous in the literature. Opponents of center theory might as well box with shadows.

Papez believed he had, in principle, resuscitated the Cannon-Bard theory of emotion. The diencephalon (mid-brain) replaced the thalamus of Cannon and the hypothalamus of Bard. Others agreed; yet there was an obvious problem: the mechanism's highest point was located not in the "neopallium" but in the "mesapallium," the underside of the cortex. Saving the theory became the task of MacLean of the Yale University School of Medicine.

MacLean's opening shot came in 1949 with his "Psychosomatic Disease and the 'Visceral Brain': Recent Developments on the Papez Theory of Emotion." The work of Herrick and Papez had made the term rhinencephalon (smell brain) obsolete. Papez had associated the old brain with emotion (without giving it a new name), and Klüver and Bucy had, two years later (1939), associated frontotemporal areas not accounted for by Papez with the emotional behavior involved in animal ferocity. MacLean enlarged Papez's circuit to include the amygdala and other parts of the frontotemporal region. He argued, also, for a new name. To MacLean's mind, animal ferocity smacks of oral behavior. And oral behavior of the ferocious variety reminded him of infants and primitives. He called this behavior "oral incorporative," just the way psychiatry was beginning to describe schizophrenia. There is little doubt that he had the psychiatrists in mind. With the ideas of orality and ferocity in hand, MacLean coined a new name, the "visceral brain."[53]

MacLean later rediscovered another name for his old brain, the "limbic system" of Herrick. In 1878 French surgeon Pierre Paul Broca had been the first to describe the system, giving it the name "limbic" because it "formed the border around" the brain stem of the rabbit. In higher animals, MacLean explained, the limbic lobe, now tucked in under the cerebral mantle, still retained its original visceral functions. It is incapable of higher (symbolic) thought and constitutes a separate brain standing over against the new brain. In higher animals the two brains can get separated, the higher losing control over the lower with the result being sham rage and catatonic schizophrenia.[54]

MacLean had preserved Cannon's vision. The decorticated animal has no subjective emotion (no feeling). This idea, central to the whole Cannon-Bard-Papez-MacLean tradition (the American mainstream) was combined with the idea that the higher centers (cortex) do the abstracting and generalizing which gets man beyond the false phenomenal world of the senses that has entrapped the old brain, to the real, abstract world of science. It is not until the cortex was formed "that one finds development of the kind of cognition that can deal coldly, analytically, and abstractly in terms of symbolic language."[55] Beneath the cortex, in the brains of the ground shrew and the rabbit, lies the murky and ferocious world of the mentally ill. MacLean described this lower realm exactly as had White: "The physician who works with 'psychosomatic' patients is frequently impressed that they share with the child and the primitive an exaggerated tendency to confuse the outside world and the inside world."[56] This was the level of the visceral, of sham rage, of the decorticated cat—behavior without feeling, machine-like behavior that chilled the observer's blood. "The animal resembles nothing so much as an idling mechanism temporarily devoid of its driver."[57] As MacLean described it, "bizarre, oral-sexual behavior."[58]

The neurophysiologists reached behind observed anatomy to impose an abstract conceptual structure—the higher-lower scheme reinforced with various localization theories. The structure was intended to give conceptual clarity to a terribly complex physical reality. It was meant to describe and explain the functioning of the anatomical masses that lay before them. Without it they had no science. But in achieving what they considered perceptual clarity, they generated the vision of sham rage, the physiologist's correlate of the Freudian id, White's horror dream of disintegrated ego boundaries, and Bleuler's schizophrenic. In the 1950s, it became fashionable to call schizophrenia "functional decortication."

For a time, neurologists felt they had the brain pretty well in hand. They felt secure enough to perform massive operations in the name of psychosurgery. Freeman and Watts cut when they thought a person was too caught up in abstractions (ideas) to act on reality. Greenblatt and Solomon cut when they saw too much emotional energy being inhibited from action and going instead into "reverberating circuits" (the invention of Herrick, Fulton, and Cobb). When ideas become so "long-circuited" — caught up in the reverberating circuits — no action can occur. The circuits become overloaded, break down into fantasy operations, absorb more and more energy until, as Freeman and Watts said, "something snaps in the head."

All this was an expression of the philosophy of the act. A person's ideas must be quickly transformed into action. If invested with too much emotion — if taken too seriously — they become more real to him than reality. Is it that ideas might become beliefs? Here, again, the model has become the other-directed person, the "Real" Miss Beauchamp.

For three generations, the mythologies of psychiatry and neurophysiology had been intertwined and mutually supporting. But in psychiatry the dynamics of perceptual interaction were causing the mythology to come unraveled. The same forces were at work in neurophysiology. It is to that subject and the continued pursuit of the Real Miss Beauchamp that we now turn.

8

CONCEPTUAL LOBOTOMY

American psychiatry entered the second half of the twentieth century in something of a bind. Its guiding theoretical structure was decomposing. Psychiatrists Karl Bowman and Milton Rose opened a 1958 symposium on schizophrenia with the statement that to "know schizophrenia is to know psychiatry." That was quite true, historically. As a science, psychiatry rode on the shoulders of the higher-lower doctrine, and the perception of the lower man was one with the perception of schizophrenia. But Bowman and Rose found no cause for satisfaction. As to the question, what is schizophrenia? they had to admit that "although some of you might venture to attempt the sort of 'explanation' demanded by the question, there is no assurance that your explanation will be understood or accepted by even a small number of your colleagues."[1] About the same time William Pious, in forming "A Hypothesis About the Nature of Schizophrenic Theory," spoke of the "enigmatic nature of the subject matter," and of the "limited usefulness and sometimes misleading connotations of available concepts and models."[2] A few years later, Robert Gibson, medical director at Sheppard and Enoch Pratt Hospital, admitted that a psychiatrist must believe in his theory to be effective, but complained this "puts us in a strange position," for as scientists "we must acknowledge the weaknesses in our system. I do not know how to avoid this."[3]

In the case of American psychiatrists, to be in doubt about schizophrenia was to be in doubt about their science. Efforts being made to discover the origins and nature of the illness were heroic. In a 1966 discussion, Semrad told of work at the Massachusetts Mental Health Center, where scientists were pursuing the problem in the fields of biochemistry, neurophysiology, pharmacology, psychopharmacology, electroencephalography, polygraphy, tissue culture, sociophysiology, psychology, community psychiatry, and clinical work—all to no avail: "Apropos the question of etiology, the answer is very simple: we do not know."[4]

Skepticism towards the fact of the disease was growing. Psychologist Eugene Gendlin at the University of Chicago charged that schizophrenia is a "catch-all category in hospitals, a label to attach to anyone who is not clearly manic-depressive, alcoholic, epileptic, or something else one can define."[5] Karl Menninger wrote in 1959 that no such disease can be proven to exist.[6] For Loren Mosher, schizophrenia had become a "wastebasket term," with "no meaning for me."[7] Thomas Szasz, in 1957, equated the term with physics' outdated idea of aether—both functioned to fill a scientific void.[8]

In the late 1950s a sense of futility hung over the field of psychiatry. Years of work with schizophrenic patients at the Forest Sanitarium led director Julius Steinfeld to conclude that there is no acceptable concept of the disease, no therapeutic approach known to work, and that the hope of cure must be abandoned.[9] In 1956, Stanley Lesse editorialized in the *American Journal of Psychotherapy* that the "most frustrating aspect of the problem" is that no particular therapy is superior to any other in helping schizophrenic patients.[10] Gene Usdin concluded in an introduction to a 1975 collection of studies on schizophrenia that "All psychiatry is facing a significant crisis today. Indeed psychiatry's very credibility is at stake." The problem was that "Schizophrenia remains a disease whose conceptual framework is fraught with confusion and uncertainty."[11]

As the 1950s waned, therapeutic fatalism spread. Johns Hopkins professor of psychiatry Jerome Frank, pointing to the fact that as many schizophrenic patients improve without therapy as with it, was led to the decisive step of abandoning theory in favor of therapeutic expediency. The important thing about therapy, he decided, is that it leads to a new self-image. His reasoning followed Harry Stack Sullivan's: the schizophrenic patient is one whose world has crumbled. "In order to function at all," wrote Frank, "everyone must impose an order and regularity on the welter of experience impinging on him." This was the new note that began to edge its way into psychiatric thought. The world outside is chaos. For the sake of mental health, order must be imposed. The ideal therapy would get the patient to "see himself as a well-equipped, competent, lovable person in a friendly, secure universe."[12] Thus, therapy became mind-cure; the art of self-deception.

The leader of this line of thought was Jules Masserman, a somewhat brilliant, Russian-born, Chicago-raised skeptic who lifted himself from obscurity on the wings of the old neurology only to emerge as psychiatry's court jester. He developed the habit of defining "insight" as "that transiently ecstatic state in which patient and therapist temporarily shared the same illusions as to the cause and cure of each other's difficulties" and was wont to call psychoanalysis an operationally effective *folie à deux*. He greeted colleagues at professional meetings with such lectures as his "Say Id Isn't So—With Music" and enjoyed relating the put-down he addressed to a meeting of the British Psychoanalytic Society when asked why American psychoanalysts end therapy after two years rather than the nine or ten that it takes in England. His response: It takes the English longer to see a joke.[13]

Masserman liked a good joke, but his skepticism ran deep. Like Frank, he concluded that mental health depends on a meaningful explanation of the world and one's role in it, and also that any such explanation is ultimately hollow. Humankind is caught in this not particularly funny dilemma. Meanings are ego defenses. Without them and the self-deception they involve, a functioning self is not possible: "Consider puny man," he wrote, "cursed since Paleolithic times with an intelligence that perceives about him a vast, chaotic, infinitely threatening universe ready at any moment to harm or destroy him." Unless he develops an intolerable anxiety, man must hold on to certain great myths—illusions, "Urdefenses"—and the job of protecting those myths has fallen on the shoulders of the psychiatrists.[14]

Without the higher-lower doctrine and the theory of emergence, without the mental health community and its related ideological trappings, psychiatry's meaningful world had crumbled. It was now the psychiatrist who was beginning to confront the specter of incomprehensibility, and the schizophrenic was its face.

A successful experimenter and a highly efficient organizer in the development of psychiatric training at Northwestern University, Masserman worked to carry on the tradition of revolt begun by Meyer, picked up by Sullivan, and continued at the Washington School of

Psychiatry. It was, after all, Sullivan who defined the "self-system" as a defense against the anxieties induced by the infant's confrontation with the world as it really is.

The institutional developments in psychiatry after World War II were less revolt than a sudden expansion and a holding action against the ambitions of the orthodox Freudians. In the process, psychiatry opened itself to a flood of new influences—such as the Washington School's point of view—which were both exhilarating and unsettling. Freudianism was no longer the locus of intellectual excitement. Once the revolutionaries, the Freudians were cast as orthodox and rigid.

The nineteenth century Association of Medical Superintendents of American Institutions for the Insane had long since given way in name to the American Psychiatric Association, and in power, more recently, to the universities. At the high-water mark of Freudian orthodoxy, there was talk of psychiatry becoming a branch of psychoanalysis. That was not to be, but by 1959 the American Psychoanalytic Association had risen to the status of independence and equality to the point of challenging the American Psychiatric Association's control of the "official" (that is, American Medical Association) examining board, the American Board of Psychiatry and Neurology. The American Psychoanalytic Association demanded its own board of examiners. The power-play failed, and one reason for the failure was the emergence of another psychoanalytic association—the Academy of Psychoanalysis—manned largely by leading academic psychiatrists together with the Washington, D.C. group loosely associated with Sullivan's Washington School. The maverick academy was organized in 1956 specifically as a counterweight to the orthodoxy of the American Psychoanalytic Association, with the purpose of opening the discipline to innovation.[15]

As American psychiatry moved well into the second half of the twentieth century, then, a rather sudden opening up to new influences occurred. The old orthodoxy—the higher-lower doctrine—was failing, and a frantic search for its replacement was begun. Mental health liberalism was awash on the rocks of schizophrenia. Without the ideology, the psychiatric professional was losing the role upon which his sense of selfhood depended.

The intellectual picture becomes one of incredible complexity as psychiatry turned to other sciences for help. For the most part these were mathematical sciences, and herein lies the real revolution in the science of the mind of recent years. A new shift in the level of abstraction was under way. To illustrate by example, I will pick up just one thread — that leading to system theory — and follow it. I will begin by inviting the reader's attention back to our old friend, sham rage.

"There is no neurophysiological contribution to the understanding of schizophrenia." (Frederick Worden, "Neurophysiological Contributions to the Understanding of Schizophrenia," 1959)

In that statement we sense something of psychiatry's anger and anguish. Just when its perceptual orientation toward the schizophrenic patient was victim to the latest turn of the dialectic and it needed all support possible from neurophysiology, its sister science backed away from the higher-lower doctrine.

I have pointed out that in the 1920s Cannon, with his "sham rage," reinvigorated the Jacksonian level theory and offered staunch support to the higher-lower mythology. He laid the foundations for Bard, Papez, MacLean, the "Yale school," and others in their attempts to localize the savage in the thalamus, hypothalamus, and, lastly, the "limbic system." "Hughlings Jackson and Head," he wrote in a 1925 article, "have pointed out that the nervous system is organized in a neural hierarchy such that primitive reactions, which might otherwise disturb the more discriminative responses of [the] higher levels, are by these repressed."[16]

In that 1925 article, Cannon first used the phrase "sham rage." He used it only in passing, and only to describe what he saw, without loading it down with metaphysical baggage. He took as his point of departure the "pseudo-affective" behavior described by the English Jacksonians, Woodward and Sherrington. He also pursued certain ideas developed in his 1915 *Bodily Changes in Pain, Hunger, Fear and Rage*, where he urged that fear and rage trigger (and register) the body's preparations for defense and flight. In 1915, Cannon took the standard position of equating the violent emotions with the primitive in man: "One needs only to glance at the history of warfare to observe that when the primitive emotions of anger and hatred are permitted full sway, men who have been considerate and thoughtful . . .

suddenly turn into infuriated savages."[17] But there was no talk of "sham rage."

In the 1925 article, in his first tentative use of "sham rage," Cannon was edging towards a radical shift in neurophysiological perspective, a shift in a certain vital sense away from the higher-lower doctrine he was defending. In that year, he announced to the Congress of American Physicians and Surgeons an idea soon to dominate neurophysiology. This was the concept of "homeostasis" (a derivative of Claude Bernard's "internal milieu"), the idea that if "a state remains steady it does so because any tendency towards change is automatically met by increased effectiveness of the factor or factors which resist the change."[18]

The coincidence of dates argues that the two ideas—"sham rage" and "homeostasis"—emerged together in Cannon's mind and leads one to suspect a relation. In fact, he saw sham rage as the obverse of homeostasis, and since homeostasis was order, sham rage was more than just a decerebrate cat's defense reactions—it was unstructure itself. And, in Cannon's own mind unstructure was the more basic: "When we consider the extreme instability of our bodily structure, its readiness for disturbance by the slightest application of external forces and the rapid onset of its decomposition as soon as favoring circumstances are withdrawn, its persistence through many decades seems almost miraculous."[19]

Seemingly without noting the distinction, Cannon spoke of homeostasis in two ways: as a system of control, and as a system of balance. In the former, the cortex figured prominently. Lower animals, he thought, lack man's homeostatic capacities because they lack the fully-developed cerebral cortex. In man, through the regulation of the internal environment, the homeostatic process frees the cortex to deal intelligently with the external environment. In their turn, the higher centers in the cortex and thalamus keep the sympathetico-adrenal system in check and sham rage inhibited. It was the mind—the subjective appreciation of emotion—that keeps violent emotion (runaway sympathetico-adrenal system) in check; sham rage was rage without mental or subjective accompaniment. The mental keeps the physical under control.[20]

So far, the higher-lower doctrine. But there was a revolutionary aspect to the homeostasis theory in that it could be construed as a balance of forces. The higher-lower doctrine was not needed. When, because of external threat, the blood needs increased sugar content and coagulation properties and the brain and muscles need faster blood circulation, the sympathetico-adrenal system will act automatically to provide them. Meanwhile, the sacral and cranial portions of the cerebro-spinal system are standing by to act in opposition to the sympathetic and bring the organism back into balance.[21] Nothing here about higher, mental control over sham rage.

I have already related the futile attempts by Bard, Papez, MacLean, and others to track down and localize sham rage. I will resume the narrative to show how, contingent on their failure, the vision of unstructure hidden in the sham rage metaphor was released and how the perception of the brain as an interacting group of gross anatomical parts—the idea of localization of function—gave way to a brain of ten billion neurons, with a hundred times more synaptic connections—a vision of infinity. I will once again urge that the project of objectification, or perceptual control, ends in generating the vision of unstructure.

When faced with the brain's unstructure, neurophysiology began to reorient itself by switching to the balance side of Cannon's idea of homeostasis, but which was in fact based on the vision of imbalance and unstructure. How structure is possible became all-absorbing. The theory of the self-organizing system began to emerge as the new scientific paradigm for many.

The announcement by Klüver and Bucy in 1939 of their discovery that removal of the temporal lobes made vicious monkeys docile, coming just when Papez was bringing some order to the diencephalic structures, was a cause for concern. Papez's scheme omitted the part—the amygdala—brought into the picture by Klüver and Bucy. The MacLean synthesis (the "limbic system")—elaborated in 1949—drew in that stray part, but there were those like MacLean's Yale laboratory coworker, Karl Pribram, who found MacLean's idea unsatisfactory. The Klüver-Bucy temporally lobectomized monkeys showed a range of behavior unexplained by MacLean. They seemed hypersexed, for one thing (to the point of scandal), and seemed to want to taste and explore everything, no matter how familiar. Certainly there was more to the amygdala than fit neatly into the rage-passivity context.[22]

Another more revolutionary blow fell with the 1949 publication of "Brain Stem Reticular Formation and Activation of the EEG," by

Guiseppe Moruzzi and Horace Magoun. It, in effect, revealed the presence of a second nervous system parallel to, and interacting with, the sensory-motor system.

Cannon's insistence that there is a subjective, and mental, side to emotion made perfect sense within the Cartesian-Jacksonian framework of a knowing mind split off from a surrounding material world. In that scheme consciousness was something qualitatively (or, ontologically) different from mere nervous excitation. Raw emotion unrefined by the thalamus, hypothalamus, or limbic system was a primitive thing to be contrasted with the higher, conscious, feelings. The Moruzzi-Magoun study showed that the truly primitive part of the nervous system was this hitherto unspecified "reticular formation" in the brain stem. It was shown to receive excitation from the sensory-motor system and, in turn, to send excitation through the thalamus and hypothalamus to all parts of the brain indiscriminately. The reticular formation was found to be nonspecific, that is, a stimulus acting on it causes the system to energize the brain as a whole.[23] Consciousness could no longer be considered a function of a "higher," something that happens to a nervous excitation as it passes some level in its ascent toward the cortex; consciousness is simply arousal, and it happens to the whole brain at once. Could there be, then, a "sham rage" of which one is not conscious?

The new development left neurophysiology in a state of conceptual shock. Donald Lindsley, a Magoun coworker, promptly (1951) outlined conclusions that had to be drawn. Emotion does not become conscious because it filters upward through the hypothalamus or thalamus but because the reticular formation has been activated. One feels more or less emotion as one is more or less aroused.[24] Loss of reticular formation activation must affect the "limbic system," or "rhinencephalon," equally with the cortex. It becomes impossible to envision the rise of the lower (the id, the unconscious) because of loss of energy to the higher. The traditional view of schizophrenia became simply unbelievable.

Because of its implications against the traditional doctrine of consciousness and control, the new discovery helped to liberate the notion of homeostasis from the higher-lower doctrine. Neurophysiologists began to envision a series of "feedback loops" (a notion got from Norbert Wiener's World War II work on finding means of feeding back error into fire-control systems) between the classical projection system and the reticular formation and even back to the receptors controlling sensory input into the nervous system.[25] Following this pattern, psychiatrists began in the 1950s to associate schizophrenia with reduced consciousness (that is, reduced activation) and presumed resulting deficiency in feedback operations: internal homeostatic imbalance or external disequilibrium—loss of feedback control over incoming stimuli.[26] S. L. Sherwood, for example, argued that an enquiry into schizophrenia "would be co-extensive with an enquiry into the modifications of consciousness," and that consciousness is a function "of the volume of information which can be continuously and simultaneously processed."[27]

Sherwood and others turned to information theory. Its originator, Claude Shannon, described information in terms of "negative entropy," or bits of order discovered against a background of unstructure, or entropy.[28] The nervous system became an "information processing system," and consciousness the degree of information processed, or, alternatively, the amount of unstructure screened out by the system. Far from regarding consciousness as a higher (human) function, J. Y. Lettvin, H. R. Maturana, W. S. McCulloch, and W. H. Pitts, in their 1959 classic "What the Frog's Eye Tells the Frog's Brain," showed that the frog's filtering process, which allows its visual system to register only five aspects of the environment, is far more powerful in this respect than man's.[29] But consciousness—the sentient life—was still tied to the notion of order. Information theory echoed Cannon's theory of homeostasis in seeing the nervous system as a dike standing against the influx of unstructure.

For many, schizophrenia was becoming the failure to stem the inflow of sensation. The literature on this soon became substantial,[30] but it was summed up in 1962 by J. W. Lovett Doust's "Consciousness in Schizophrenia as a Function of Peripheral Microcirculation," with the conclusion that the schizophrenic defect is the inability to "establish relevance for the input signals."[31]

At this point I wish to insert a disclaimer. By no means did all neurophysiologists desert the Jacksonian standard. Besides the Freudians, one might mention the (1950-1960) Tulane Project and the psychiatric conclusions growing from it made by Russell Monroe in his *Episodic Behavioral Disorders* (1970).[32] Monroe made Hughlings Jackson's description of the epileptic the explanation for most of the individual and social disorders of our age. One might also mention R. L. Isaacson's 1974, *The Limbic System*, in which names—Graven Image, Lethe, Guru—were given to each of the presumed functions of MacLean's three brain tiers.[33]

Meanwhile, some higher-lower speculation developed around "split-brain" research.[34] Evidence suggests that speech and writing are processed best in the left (dominant) hemisphere, and nonverbal stimuli, in the right. Based on this, the speculative hypothesis emerged that the left hemisphere is the more analytic of the two, specializing in breaking sensory patterns down into their parts, while the right is more holistic, registering the patterns and building them into a gestalt.[35] Data from one of their patients led neurologist Michael Gazzaniga and his colleagues to hypothesize that the verbal left hemisphere puts into words, thus into consciousness, what the right hemisphere does (in overt behavior) and feels.[36] This sort of theorizing led a psychologist, Julian Jaynes, to attempt a full-scale revival of the higher-lower mythology.[37]

Also, not all of those for whom the Cannon-Bard-Papez-MacLean structure exploded into the unstructure of the ten billion neurons gave up hope that by tracing neural pathways a means would be found to rebuild the vision of a brain composed of gross anatomical parts interacting in the fashion of Newtonian mechanics. This group became known as the "pathway neurophysiologists." Perhaps the most accurate statement to be made about the state of neurophysiology as it entered the 1970s was University of Oslo Professor A. Brodal's that "as research progresses it becomes increasingly difficult to separate functionally different regions of the brain," and that "the fragments of knowledge cannot yet be put together in a meaningful way."[38]

Now, a word concerning the decline of the Jackson-Cannon-Bard-MacLean paradigm. My first point was that sham rage was (like the unconscious, and schizophrenia) a metaphor that hid the vision of the brain as unstructure. The attempt to localize sham rage, first in the lower and then in a particular anatomical part of the lower, was both an affirmation of the higher-lower dogma and an attempt to put the brain into the conceptual scheme of Newtonian mechanics—the linear action of objects upon one another in an orderly and measurable way. At that time the neurophysiologists were still dealing with phenomenal objects—concrete individual things that appear before the senses and that, unfortunately for science, have the tendency of all concrete individual things to become infinite in their complexity.

Light is shed on Cannon's "homeostasis" when put in the context of the "self-control trap," that is, the dialectic of objectification. The self-control trap of late nineteenth-century literature expressed fear of spiraling into disintegration (savagery), as one pressed onward with self-control and progressively used up energy needed for control. It was a recognition on the level of anxious premonition of the dialectic of objectification. Resolution came in the idea, expressed by Hall, of putting behind one's isolated (phenomenal) individuality by merging into community. This constituted a step in abstraction, from the phenomenal level where one is faced by the infinite individual (thus, the residue) to the logical level of Holt where behavior is defined by the logical calculus.

The dialectic expressed in "homeostasis" was but an extension of the one voiced in psychiatry. When the cat goes into sham rage, the investigator loses perceptual control (predictability) over the animal. Cannon was quick to generalize from the cat's behavior to the savagery lurking in all men. By localizing the unpredictable in an anatomical part, it might be contained and rendered finite. Each successive step towards localization turned out to be a step toward discovering the futility of the localizing exercise. With each step, the brain is seen to be more complex and more defiant of explanation. Soon, given a boost by Moruzzi and Magoun, the brain exploded out of its system of concrete anatomical parts into randomness — 10^{10} (or more) neurons with an infinite number of synaptic interconnections (the number of synapses on individual neurons range from one to 80,000), and the potential for perhaps an infinite number of possible instantaneous brain states.[39] Faced with this collapse into the infinite, there emerged once again the tendency to shift levels of abstraction, from the phenomenal realm of the (apparently) concrete individual to the mathematical-logical level of systems theory. Homeostasis becomes the system, sham rage its collapse. At that point sham rage became for neuro-physiology what "oral incorporation" became for psychiatry, the loss of (ego) boundaries between the observer and the observed.

There is much to suggest that systems theory is the historical successor to mental health liberalism as an ideology of the middle-class professional. It is still too much a part of the present to hope for more than a partial and impressionistic account of its scope and influence, but without some attempt my story will be incomplete.[40]

We are said to be living in a postindustrial age.[41] It is possible that systems theory will take its place as the postindustrial ideology. Certainly, systems theorists self-consciously see their approach as the postindustrial age science. Except for its heavy emphasis on Cannon's homeostasis, systems theorists have turned to the language and concepts of modern technology for their theoretical premises.[42]

During World War II, Norbert Wiener assumed the job of solving the problem of shooting at fast-moving targets such as airplanes, something manually-controlled weapons could not accomplish. His solution was the syncro-servo mechanism, and from his solution he developed the philosophy of cybernetics: self-controlling systems operate on the principle of feeding back error in to the input. Wiener's *Cybernetics* (1948) and *The Human Use of Human Beings* (1954) thus stand as primary documents in systems theory history. Right beside them stand the works of W. Ross Ashby (*An Introduction to Cybernetics* of 1956, and *Design for a Brain*, 1952), and W. Gray Walter's *The Living Brain* (1953). Through Ashby and Walter, cybernetics was expanded into automaton (robot) theory and artificial intelligence. Then, by interpreting feedback in terms of information and by giving information a mathematical basis, the field of artificial intelligence was given a large boost. The basic document here is Claude Shannon and Warren Weaver's *The Mathematical Theory of Information* (1949).[43]

And, of course, the central element in modern technology from which systems theory drew was computer technology. The computer's advance in performing functions previously considered the exclusive domain of the human brain gave artificial intelligence theory its appeal. And the close parallel between the performances of the computer and the brain made cybernetics and information theory seem explanatory for neurophysiology.[44]

The widespread use of systems theory as technique in postindustrial society argues its centrality for ideology. "Operational research and its offspring, systems analysis," wrote Lilienfeld, "are the most important of the systems approaches, having had a direct impact on American government and policymaking at the federal, state, and municipal levels." Lilienfeld listed the fields of transportation, waste disposal, health, education, social welfare, crime control, traffic control, and food supply as areas in which systems theory has been tried and pointed to the disciplines of communication theory, systems engineering, management science, game and decision theory as offspring.

For many, the discovery of coding in DNA and protein molecules was a giant boost for the systems theory approach. One result was the new genetics of Alfred Emerson, Theodosius Dobzhansky, and Ernest Meyer. It also led to a reanalysis of evolutionary theory in the hands of Jacques Monod and Gregory Bateson in terms of "stochastic" systems, wherein self-maintaining systems are thought to evolve by creatively assimilating chance or random inputs.[45]

Two of the leading names to pick up on systems theory in the social sciences were perhaps Talcott Parsons and Gordon Allport. Both came to systems theory in mid-career. Parsons tells us ("On Building a Social System Theory: A Personal History," 1977) that the theory provides a bridge between human societies and the biological world, while Allport saw systems theory as providing the framework for bringing behaviorism, ego-psychology, self-actualization theory, and ego-defense theory under one roof.[46] Meanwhile, the work done in the name of psychology to bring cognitive processes into line with information-processing theory and thus into systems theory was nearly endless.[47] In the science of cognitive processes, at least, systems theory became normative in the 1970s.

Postindustrial technology gave us, in systems theory, a new vocabulary. Did it, as nearly all its advocates believe, give us a new, postmechanistic science? The arguments in favor of the proposition are, first, that by looking at the whole system, rather than merely at the parts, systems theory avoids the linear cause-effect approach of traditional science, and, second, that by discovering systems at each level—from particle physics through chemistry, biology, social groups, on out to the universe—isomorphisms between levels can be discovered, thus bringing all phenomena under one unified science—general systems theory.

The originator of the general systems theory idea was Ludwig von Bertalanffy, whose special interest was psychiatry. It was von Bertalanffy's contention that the mechanistic model of man (that is, behaviorism) has the potential of turning us all into robots. A holistic, or organismic model (systems theory) will return the human sciences to the humanistic vision. But as we listen to von Bertalanffy, we hear echoes of the past: "Personality is not a robot; but in mental disease when spontaneity is impaired, the patient may *become* an S–R automaton."[48]

There is another reason for wondering whether systems theory is not merely a new and perhaps more sophisticated mechanism. Systems theory emphasizes that it is the system or program that governs, for example, the machine. We learn to understand the machine not by tracing the sequence of cause-effect through the moving parts but by looking at the structure programmed into it. In this argument, we hear echoes of Holt's declaration for logical form. Through one's behavior one returns to a means-end world, fulfilling one's form (program). One enters the realm governed by the logical calculus and leaves behind one's lower, mechanistic self.

For a time the systems theorists believed that the logical calculus of the philosophers was the means of freeing us from mechanism. Warren McCulloch and Walter Pitts attempted to bring this intuition to the working of "neural nets" in the brain. Their 1943 "A Logical Calculus of the Ideas Imminent in Nervous Activity"[49] became an acknowledged forerunner of artificial intelligence theory. They tried to show how systems of neurons ("neural nets") may operate by mathematical logic. The firing of neurons, separately or in combination, was argued to constitute a (logical) proposition to succeeding neurons, which, in their turn, act to confirm the proposition by firing or to reject it by not firing. Coming back to his theory some years later, McCulloch sadly admitted he had failed to go beyond a linear cause-effect sequence in his description of events.[50] When embodied in material events such as neurons, logic becomes mechanistic.

Gregory Bateson, the anthropologist who became famous for his "double-bind" theory of schizophrenia, has shown where the trouble lay. When one tries to describe the operation of a simple machine in terms of logic, one always ends with a logical paradox (a contradiction) — while the machine goes on its merry, mechanistic way.[51]

So the project, suggested in the von Bertalanffy quote above, to restate the higher-lower doctrine in terms of a post-mechanistic logical calculus as the higher and mechanism as the lower (Holt's project), came to naught. But the early attempts, such as McCulloch's and Pitts's, formed a bridge that guided many of those bred in the higher-lower doctrine into systems theory once the higher-lower collapsed.

The bridge, the transition stage, is strongly evident in one of the most important of psychiatry's systems theory documents, Karl Menninger's *Vital Balance*. Like Holt before him (whose *Freudian Wish* he called a classic), Menninger set out to restate Freud in systems theory terms. But this was a later Freud than the one Holt dealt with—the Freud of the "death instinct." Pure destructiveness—the oral incorporation vision—has taken equal place with the life forces, the libido. In Menninger's hands, the life instinct becomes the organismic drive towards systems-maintenance, with the ego a special subsystem which, like a machine's governor, acts to preserve organization. On the other hand, there is the death instinct, or aggressiveness—the constant tendency towards disorganization.[52]

Again, the *Vital Balance* was a transition document. The higher and the lower can be vaguely identified in it, with organization (balance) as the higher and aggressiveness as the lower. But one might as justly identify the higher with the ego, the governor, and the maintainer of balance. And it is difficult to absolutely identify aggressiveness with the lower because it has become an equal partner without which the life instinct in its drive for order could not be creative. Without the struggle between two opposing forces, there is loss of balance, leading either to chaos or to stultifying order.

What was new in Menninger's work was that disorganization or chaos was no longer localized either in a part of the body or in a lower self. In the *Vital Balance*, chaos has achieved ontological status. It is no longer residue.

A second transitional document, of perhaps equal importance with the *Vital Balance*, was the report of four conferences brought together in the early 1950s by neurophysiologist Roy Grinker to discuss the possibility of a unified theory of behavior. Grinker was long associated with the Institute for Psychosomatic and Psychiatric Research and Training of Michael Reese Hospital in Chicago. The American psychosomatic movement had roots sunk deep in the "psychobiology" and "organismic" approach of the Jelliffe-White-Meyer circle.[53] The fact that "organismic" became an alternate term for "systems" indicates something of the directness of the progression in neuropsychiatry from the White circle to systems theory.

The report of those four conferences, *Toward a Unified Theory of Human Behavior*, published in 1956, became one of the two leading source books for general systems theory.[54] Its participants ranged from neurophysiology through anthropology. Talcott Parsons was present, as were David and Anatol Rapoport. Philosophy was represented by Charles Morris, and Pavlovian psychology by Howard Liddell. If one theme ran through the discussions, it was this: chaos is primary.

In another place, Masserman had concluded that the "self-system" is a defense mechanism against universal chaos. At the second conference, held in April 1953, Grinker's conclusion was even more radical. Every function of every structure—be it a human organism or a social system—exists to defend that structure against chaos: "I speak of [a system's] function as integrative, or in other words, opposed to disintegration—it is the capacity to maintain or defend itself against randomness."[55]

Late-nineteenth-century genteel neurology had begun to feel itself confronted by a growing class of degenerates, whose energy resources were dissipated and who threatened to carry society down with them into savagery. Now, in the 1950s, following the new technology, the words had changed. Energy gave way to information. Decreased information was defined as increased randomness. So, now, the mentally ill were no longer to be considered carriers of a disease germ or alien agency. Now they were to be considered as carriers of randomness. Neurophysiologist James Toman told the conference that the difference between insect societies and human society is the vastly increased potential in the latter for disorganization. The mentally ill become barometers for measuring the degree of disorganization present, and, moreover, "the bizarre behavior or inability to function in a useful way of even a few individuals can potentially have cataclysmic consequences for the many."[56]

We surmise that for Toman schizophrenia was a contagious disease. How can that be so? The answer lies in the new conceptualization of its nature. It was no longer loss of energy but loss of information. Loss of energy in the patient does not affect the psychiatrist, but loss of information in the person observed directly affects the observer. So the shift from energy to information reflected more than a shift from steam engine technology to computer; it reflected the new vulnerability of the position of the observer. He has been drawn into the system. When it disintegrates he does too.

A second assumption of profound significance that ran through the four conferences involved the universal use of the term "personality" and the absence of any concept of self or selfhood. Loss of self or disintegration of the self-system had always been a basic assumption about schizophrenia. The systems theory conferees spoke of the "individual" quite often, but in a new way. In their minds, the social sciences of the past had falsely pitted the individual against some preexisting ("reified") system—the social system, the political system, or the economic system. That had made for a dualism that systems theory wished to transcend.

Conferee Lawrence Frank made it clear that the true progression is from biology (the infant) to socialized personality (the adult).[57] The "organism-personality," as Frank called it, makes the transition directly from one system (biological) to another (social). One result of this approach was the abandonment of the higher-lower doctrine, a doctrine that involves selves. Frank's biological system simply becomes a subsystem of the social, not a lower pitted against a higher.

A second and vital aspect of Frank's approach was the omission of the subjective or psychological dimension of the individual, just as the homeostasis-chaos interpretation of Cannon's theory had no place for a higher, controlling subjectivity. The new position was voiced by a somewhat perplexed Roy Grinker when he noted that systems theory jumps directly from somatic description to social interaction description and back, leaving out the psychological.[58] In systems theory, the patient's ideas became irrelevant.

What was involved here was a shift from the medical model in psychiatry to what psychiatrist Edgar Auerswald termed the "ecological" approach.[59] Auerswald related the reactions of two therapists to a twelve-year-old inner city girl who was in the habit of running away from home. Because she seemed abstracted, the traditionalist psychotherapist labeled her a schizophrenic and ordered her institutionalized. The systems theory psychiatrist, on the other hand, after speaking with the girl's mother, teachers, social workers, and the police, decided that a less disorganized home life was the answer. Had he gotten his way, the girl's family and community relations would have been altered. In his mind, she would have been reprogrammed.

The case interests us because not once did the systems psychiatrist interview the girl herself; not once did he attempt to explore her ideas or her subjectivity. Don Jackson, one-time director of the Palo Alto Mental Research Institute, tells us why: "We view symptoms, defenses, character structure, and personality as terms describing the individual's typical interactions which occur in response to a particular interpersonal context, rather than as intrapsychic entities."[60] Systems theory labels the individual a biological entity until he enters into interaction with others in some sort of group. At that point group interaction both develops a pattern particular to that group and draws the individual into the program constituted by that pattern. The individual transcends mere biology to the extent that he is programmed.

From the discussion, it is possible to isolate four points characteristic of this new direction for neuropsychiatry, systems theory. First, there is the presentment of chaos; unstructure takes the same ontological status as order. It is no longer mere residue. On the one hand, systems theorists picture a world in which subsystems, systems, and suprasystems pyramid upward and outward from the atomic level to envelop the universe in a sort of modern-day version of the Great Chain of Being. Order incorporates the world. On the other hand, structure is seen as a tiny island adrift in the great, universal ocean of randomness—entropy. This dichotomy of vision is non-Cartesian.

Second, the observer's position has become problematic. He knows that as he enters into a relation with the patient, he is entering a group system of interactions. He knows that as this new group develops, he, as well as the patient, will either be newly programmed or will be thrown into a mutual state of disorganization. Either way, the interactions will become part of him.

Third, there is no longer a search for the Real Miss Beauchamp because selves as such are no longer believed in. The notion that a person has a true self for which therapist and patient search has become nonsense. But this does not mean that the Real Miss Beauchamp has made her exit from our story.

Fourth, ideas (subjectivity) have become irrelevant. The old psychiatry, in its analysis of the patient's ideas, reflected the American inner-directed past, a past when the person was identified with his ideas. In the Real Miss Beauchamp, Prince created an other-directed person, and it was she who became the ideal for mental health liberalism. A person was to be defined not by ideas but by actions. In the process of creating the Real Miss Beauchamp, Prince created himself as professional—a person for whom ideas are manipulative tools. The inner-directed person, whose ideas were guiding beliefs, no longer defined either the doctor or patient. Systems theory merely reflects the fact of the other-directed person.

CONCLUSION

In his *Eclipse of Reason*, Max Horkheimer tells us that corporate industrialism disorganizes the subjectivity of those it makes its objects of organization. Miss Beauchamp was a victim of this process, but so was Morton Prince. At the beginning, both were genteel — products of the genteel mix between traditional and inner-directed controls. But neither of these sets of controls could withstand the dialectic of objectification.

William James was the victim of a fading self — disorganized subjectivity. The doxological conceptual mapping was organized around the perception of a "self" (an "essence") that was directly seen in the overt behavior of others. But behavior must be responsive — ends must be visible in the means — if the self, the essence, is to be seen. James's world was no longer responsive to him, and his own selfhood was implicated in his growing uncertainty as to how to respond to others.

As traditional life breaks down and one's emotions are no longer channeled by group ceremony, they must be handled individually. In the inner-directed individual, emotions are controlled and directed by strong belief systems. Darwin's theory of natural selection brought biology into a mechanistic frame for James and his contemporaries. Scientific naturalism became queen, and belief systems came under her reign. But for James, the mechanistic frame dissolved under the positivism of Chauncy Wright. Beliefs became mere beliefs. James found himself expending his time and energy trying to deal with emotions unlinked to traditional forms or to a strong belief system. So much time and energy went into emotional control that he decided he, along with so many of the genteel, was a victim of neurasthenia.

We can say that James's subjective unity was shattered. Lacking the ties of tradition and the guidance of a strong belief system, he could no longer be certain of his response patterns. He no longer had himself under perceptual control. His selfhood was fading.

The genteel stood at the crossroads. James was one of the first to decide that ideas are not truths; they are guides to behavior. Would they be used to open one up to immediate experience, and perhaps through that sting to the treasures of beauty as well as to the evils the world holds, or would they be used in the attempt to coerce the world into predictability? In the latter case, ideas would become tools of the technician, and one's subjective unity would become hostage to the efficacy of one's manipulative powers.

Morton Prince's subjective unity was challenged by Miss Beauchamp's failure to respond as expected. Miss Beauchamp's subjective unity was shattered once she accepted Prince's theory of her many selves. On entering their seven-year relation, both were genteel. One suspects that on leaving, both were other-directed. Prince achieved perceptual control by adopting the techniques of manipulation and the role of doctor. Miss Beauchamp achieved selfhood by submitting to those techniques and by assuming the role of patient.

The doxological mapping reflected the experience of perceptual control. Violation of perceptual clarity was violation of the doxological and was registered as absence of self. When a naughty smile flashed across Miss Beauchamp's sad countenance, her selfhood faded for Prince. By imagining "Sally," the demonic, he established a cause, and in so doing shifted mappings from the design of the doxological to the cause-effect of the mechanistic. The reconceptualization brought with it a different perception. The mechanistic mapping made Prince experience Miss Beauchamp as a mere machine, an automaton.

The new conceptual mapping did not eliminate residue, it only generated a new one. Sally's behavior was residue to the doxological mapping; the dream was residue to the mechanistic. Miss Beauchamp became a dreaming-machine, a somnambulist. In the mechanistic mapping, one retreats to the position of observer, but one is facing an automaton over which there is no control. The psychiatric experience with the schizophrenic following World War II shows how the response patterns to this experience became problematic. One's subjective unity is once again threatened. The dream metaphor expressed Prince's loss of perceptual control over himself.

Thus the project for mental health liberalism was set: bring the dream into the public reality. This project defined the mental health liberal's ideal community.

The stage was set for paradox and contradiction. The patient's dream was a disguise for the psychiatrist's loss of perceptual control. The analysis of the dream turns out to be the disguised analysis by the analyst of himself. As he analyzed the dream, he moved ever further into the mechanistic mapping, thus intensifying his own perceptual response to mechanism—his own loss of perceptual control over himself. The more he analyzed the patient into the mechanistic mapping, the more his own responses became disorganized and the more the dream grew in power. The psychiatrist expressed this as the rise of the unconscious within himself. He was being plunged into the non-Cartesian dualism.

The Real Miss Beauchamp was one side of the non-Cartesian dualism and finally found her mapping in systems theory. However, so long as the metaphors held, the mechanistic mapping held for the lower, and it was still possible to think of the Real Miss Beauchamp as an emergent out of mechanism.

If conceptual mappings had lives of their own, we might think of them as constantly testing their own limits. This testing generates its own residue, and the residual category is then made part of the mapping—Sally becomes cause to Miss Beauchamp's effect; the savage becomes cause to the morally insane person's effect, and so forth. But the residue stands in violation of the mapping—in Sally, in the savage, and in the dream, the mapping is put in the position of containing its own violation. This is the stuff of paradox, and we might say that if conceptual mappings had lives of their own and test their own limits, the limits are set by paradox. In the case of the mechanistic mapping, at least, the paradox was played out in the dialectic of objectification.

Mechanism contrasts the observer with the observed. In the Cartesian dualism, which expresses this split, subject is pitted against object. The problem for logic becomes this: if the Cartesian dualism is real it must belong to one side or the other of itself. The dualism itself must either be merely subjective or it must belong to objective reality. If the latter is true, the object world must incorporate subjectivity within it. Put another way, the observed must contain the observer—the situation described by Heisenberg's indeterminacy.

In the paradox, the mechanistic mapping has reached its limit. In psychological terms, the paradox expresses the felt dissolution of the psychiatrist's ego boundaries. The distinction between in-here and out-there collapses for the psychiatrist into a non-Cartesian world. The moment of truth for the mechanistic mapping of the insane (the residue) arrived with the attempt to apply psychotherapy to the waking dream—the schizophrenic. In attempting to analyze the dream as though it characterized the patient, the psychiatrist was objectifying his own subjectivity.

In watching his own erratic behavior, the psychiatrist became object to himself. In projecting the resulting perceptual confusion onto the patient as dream, the psychiatrist restored his own subjectivity (subjective unity). He now had his mapping. So long as the dream metaphor held, the subject-object mapping (and the mechanism it supported) was possible. When the dream metaphor failed, the subject-object dichotomy failed with it. Within the context of the mechanistic mapping, the psychiatrist's ego boundaries depended upon the dream metaphor; when it failed, those ego boundaries collapsed with it. This was expressed in the experience of "oral incorporation."

But was the dream an expression of the psychiatrist's subjectivity, or was it an expression of residue—that part of the outside world which violated his conceptual mapping? It was both, and it was neither. At this point, the terms "subject" and "object" begin to lose their usefulness, and we must consider shifting to the terms "private domain" and "public reality." In making this shift, we recognize that the public reality of any group is defined by a shared conceptual mapping. "Self" and "essence" were public reality under the doxological mapping. Nineteenth-century mechanism turned to measurement and linear cause-effect sequences for its public reality. Mental health liberalism proposed to save the doxological as the public reality for the sane by establishing mechanism as the public reality for the insane.

In the process of defining its public reality in mechanistic terms, science since Galileo defined subjectivity as the repository for all that did not fit measurement and cause-effect sequences. Subjectivity, it was said, was composed of the "secondary qualities" of things. That which is subjective, it was said, is that which is private. That which is subjective was also characterized as that which is mental.

Thus the subject-object dichotomy became an essential part of the mechanistic mapping. That which did not conform to the mechanistic public reality—that which was private—was said to be subjective and mental. That which did not fit the public reality was residual, and in bringing the residue into the mapping itself, the mapping was made to harbor its own violation.

When the psychiatrist brought the patient into the mechanistic realm (for example, by identifying the demonic as cause) his own responses became disorganized and unpredictable. His reaction (and here we are back to the dialectic) was to objectify those responses. In effect, he began to establish what the psychiatrists call "ego boundaries" between himself and his own behavior, and when he did so, his ego boundaries (defined by the subject-object dualism) began to crumble. This is the point at which the dream metaphor had its beginning. By projecting his perceptual disorganization as the patient's dream, the psychiatrist took the pressure off the Cartesian dualism for the time. The dream was the subject-object paradox itself, or, rather, its metaphorical statement. It (and the schizophrenic) was the embodiment of the non-Cartesian dualism into which the psychiatrist was being thrown when trying to establish ego boundaries between himself and his own behavior.

The dream, then, was both the product of mechanism and a residual category to the Cartesian dualism. The attempt to analyze the schizophrenic was the project of bringing the dream into the public reality, making room in the Cartesian dualism for its own violation.

But the dream was mind and could not be integrated back into the material, causal sequence, which was described as public reality by mechanism. Subsequent events can be described in two ways: first, as the playing out of the perceptual dialectic, in which the dream (the non-Cartesian dualism) swelled and swallowed up the psychiatrist; second, in terms of the resulting shift in levels of abstraction.

To take the first case. The dream metaphor failed in post-World War II psychiatry partly because of the demise of the savage in the hands of Sullivan. The dream was, after all, the savage dream, effect to the savage cause. It was the savage as cause that helped tie the dream into the objective world of cause and effect. Once severed of its relation with the savage, the dream's localization "out there" became problematic; it became "incorporative," breaking down the line between observer and observed. In Sullivan's hands, the unconscious (the "not me") lost its connotation as dream and became merely the disintegration of the patient's world. Others, like Masserman and Frank, followed, accepting Sullivan's point that the chaos of the "not me" is a true description of the world. It was the psychiatrist's loss of structure (concomitant with the failure of his mythology) that spelled the end of the dream metaphor.

When the dream metaphor failed, the private domain or the residue could no longer be dismissed as subject. It broke into the open with an ontological status equal to the public reality; which is to say that it was no longer even private. Now chaos (the old private) and order (the old public) stood side by side in a non-Cartesian dualism, freed from connotations of subject and object.

Miss Beauchamp, once made "real," could have no private life. She must be either chaos or order.

To take the second case. The dream could be saved for the public reality in only one way, by changing the public reality—by changing the mapping. By shaking the causal chain free from the mind-matter dualism, by making it neither mental nor physical but neutral (behavior), and by redefining the dream into the same neutral terms (Holt's "repressed tendencies to act"), dream and the public reality could be reconciled.

But, with the shift in mapping, there was no reason for saving the dream metaphor. Interaction between two human beings (Prince and Sally), or between psychiatrist and dreaming-machine (Prince and BI), gave way to manipulation and controlled response (Prince and the Real Miss Beauchamp).

This step in abstraction was the one taken by systems theory. The relation between observer and observed became that which held between the mathematician and his equation in algebra. The equation works no matter who performs operations on it—it is the public reality. But the equation has nothing to do with sense experience, and nor does the system.

In neurophysiology, the moment of truth for nineteenth-century mechanism came with the failure to localize sham rage and thus establish a mechanistic mapping for the brain. Sham rage had been taken as evidence of the savage, thus giving the savage a place in the causal chain of events, the cause of compulsions and other insane behaviors.

But sham rage defied localization, and since it made sense as the collapse of homeostasis or order, a shift in mappings resulted. Sham rage was for neurophysiology what "oral incorporation" was for psychiatry, the collapse of nineteenth-century mechanism and a shift in the relation between observer and the observed.

Systems theory (a new mechanism?) constituted a next step in abstraction. The model was still the machine, but it was no longer the causal chain of events described by the working parts. It was now the (self-regulating) pattern of which the working parts are the expression. People were still thought to interact, but they simply carry out a program inherent in the particular group. It is not the individual as a self who is real, nor is it the group. It is the program, the pattern, the harmony, and the order expressed in the working of the group.

System, though it has acquired great sophistication in cybernetic theory, information theory, and so forth, is essentially Holt's version of the higher. The old lower has lost its metaphors and become disorder or chaos. On the one hand, all existence is described in terms of subsystem, system, and suprasystem, no matter whether we make our cut at the atomic level, the chemical level, and so forth, on up to the universe itself. On the other hand, order is seen to be a tiny island in a vast ocean of entropy.

But how do matters now stand in the search for the Real Miss Beauchamp?

At present, the matter of mental illness reduces to whether a given person is programmable. If so, a behaviorist is called in to develop a program. If not (if the person is hostile, aggressive, and generally unmanageable) it becomes a medical matter and a medical person — psychiatrist or neurologist — is brought in armed with a variety of chemical substances, hopefully to restore homeostasis (that is, programmability).

In systems theory, we go from the medical model to the ecological model. We no longer see people as tradition-directed or inner-directed. They are part of the system. The other-directed person has become the model of reality itself. The medical model (in the higher-lower tradition) was largely a carry-over from the inner-directed model of man, when it was thought that a person is defined by his beliefs. It was incumbent upon the psychiatrist to interest himself in those beliefs. The systems theory psychiatrist, on the other hand, feels little need to explore the patient's private reality, because no private reality exists for systems theory. The Sally vision is dead. It is no longer conceivable that one might march to a different drummer. Either one is in step or there is chaos. We are reminded of a military formation.

The question of how matters stand with Miss Beauchamp largely turns on how matters stand with Sally. So far in this conclusion, for the sake of convenience, I have spoken as if the mechanistic mapping was sole successor to the doxological. But this was not so, there was the less pronounced theme of vitalism or materialism.

We see Sally as psychiatry's explanation for residual events. But the striking thing about her was that she was experienced first hand, she was real for Prince. She made the mechanistic public reality possible by serving as cause, but in herself she was Prince's private reality— immediately experienced phenomena that did not fit the Real Miss Beauchamp. She served the mental health liberals as an alternative vision—the creative child (or libido, and so forth)—in her active resistance to the physician's expectations and manipulations and to his detached objectivity as well. She approached him through the seams of his mappings, beckoning him to step out from behind his security and to face her infinitude.

If each individual around me is considered infinite in her or his complexity, then my perceptions of each and all must be private, for I will select aspects no one else will select. This book has described the confrontation that took place with the infinite, and the step-by-step retreat out of the private domain into the public reality.

NOTES

CHAPTER 1. THE NINETEENTH-CENTURY BACKGROUND

1. Norman Dain, *Concepts of Insanity in the United States, 1789-1865* (New Brunswick, N.J.: Rutgers University Press, 1964), p. 5.

2. Gerald Grob, *The State and the Mentally Ill: A History of Worcester State Hospital in Massachusetts, 1830-1920* (Chapel Hill: University of North Carolina Press, 1966), p. 8. See, however, the dissenting view of Andrew Scull, "Madness and Segregative Control: The Rise of the Insane Asylum," *Social Problems* 24 (February 1977):337-51, who argues that the asylum movement grew out of the rise of capitalism and consequent transformation of economic relations into purely market relations. Economic relations were divested of personal ties and the traditional relations between rich and poor sundered.

3. George Rosen, *Madness in Society: Chapters in the Historical Sociology of Mental Illness* (London: Routledge and Kegan Paul, 1968).

4. Michel Foucault, *Madness and Civilization: A History of Insanity in the Age of Reason*, trans. Richard Howard (New York: Pantheon Books, 1968).

5. Grob, *The State and the Mentally Ill*, p. 56; Dain, *Concepts of Insanity*, p. 89.

6. See Amariah Brigham's *Observations on the Influence of Religion upon the Health and Physical Welfare of Mankind* (Boston: Marsh, Capen, and Lyon, 1835), and *Inquiry Concerning the Diseases and Functions of the Brain and the Nerves* (New York: George Adlard, 1840); and Isaac Ray, *Mental Hygiene* (Boston: Tichnor and Fields, 1863).

7. See Richard Bushman's *From Puritan to Yankee: Character and the Social Order in Connecticut, 1690-1765* (Cambridge, Mass.: Harvard University Press, 1967).

8. See Philip Greven's *The Protestant Temperament: Patterns of Child Rearing, Religious Experience, and the Self in Early America* (New York: Alfred Knopf, 1977).

9. Thomas Arnold, *Observations on the Nature, Kinds, Causes, and Prevention of Insanity*, 2d ed. (London: Richard Phillips, 1806), 1:163.

10. Isaac Ray, "Moral Insanity" (1861), in *Contributions to Mental Pathology* (Boston: Little, Brown and Co., 1873), p. 108.

11. See Arthur Fink, *Causes of Crime: Biological Theories in the United States* (Philadelphia: University of Pennsylvania Press, 1938); Mark Haller, *Eugenics. Hereditarian Attitudes in American Thought, 1870-1930* (New Brunswick, N.J.: Rutgers University Press, 1963); Georges Genil-Perrin, *Histoire des origins et de l'évolution de l'idée de dégénérescence en médecine* (Paris: A. Leclerc, 1913); Alfred Lindsmith and Yale Levin, "The Lombrosian Myth in Criminology," *American Journal of Sociology* 42 (March 1937):653-71.

12. Benjamin Rush, *Medical Inquiry and Observations upon the Diseases of the Mind* (Philadelphia: Kimber and Richardson, 1812), pp. 27, 150; Philippe Pinel, *A Treatise of Insanity*, trans. D. D. Davis (Sheffield, England: Printed by W. Todd, 1806), p. 12; Jean Esquirol, *Des Passions, Considérées comme Causes, Symptômes, et Moyens curatifs de l'Aliénation mentale* (Paris: Didot Jeune, 1805), p. 21. See the appendix of Karl Menninger et al., *The Vital Balance: The Life Process in Mental Health and Illness* (New York: Viking Press, 1963), pp. 419-89, for a comprehensive historical summary of psychiatric nosologies from Hippocrates to the present. Rush, Pinel, and Esquirol are pictured as sharing in a humanitarian reaction against multiplying disease entities. They largely abandoned classification for clinical description of the patient. See also Ilza Veith, "Psychiatric Nosology: From Hippocrates to Kraepelin," *American Journal of Psychiatry* 114 (November 1957):385-91.

13. John Conolly, *An Inquiry Concerning the Indications of Insanity, with Suggestions for the Better Protection and Care of the Insane* (London: Printed for John Taylor, 1830), pp. 166-67.

14. James Cowles Prichard, *A Treatise on Insanity and Other Disorders Affecting the Mind* (Philadelphia: Sherwood, Gilbert, and Piper, 1837), 21-22.

15. Rosen, *Madness in Society*, p. 10; Grob, *The State and the Mentally Ill*, p. 52; Eric Carlson and Norman Dain, "The Meaning of Moral Insanity," *Bulletin of the History of Medicine* 36 (March-April 1962):132-33; Dain, *Concepts of Insanity*, p. 10.

16. J. J. Quinn, "Homicidal Insanity—The Case of Nancy Farrer," *American Journal of Insanity* 12 (April 1856): 334 (hereafter *AJI*).

17. Pliny Earle, *Memoirs of Pliny Earle, M.D.*, ed. F. B. Sanborn (Boston: Damsell and Upham, 1898), pp. 221-22.

18. Isaac Ray, "The Causes of Insanity" (1864), in *Contributions*, p. 53; John Butler, Hartford Retreat Annual *Report*, quoted in *AJI*, 13 (April 1857):330; P. Boileau De Castelnau, "On Instantaneous Insanity, Considered in a Medico-Legal Point of View," *AJI* 9 (July 1852):9.

19. Isaac Ray, "An Examination of the Objections to the Doctrine of Moral Insanity," *AJI*, 18 (October 1861):115; Ray, *Contributions*, p. 102; Butler, Hartford Retreat, *AJI* 13 (April 1857):330; *Report* of the Mount Hope Institution (1848), excerpted in *AJI* 11 (January 1855):265; A. O. Kellogg, "Considerations on the Reciprocal Influence of the Physical Organization and Mental Manifestations," *AJI* 11 (January 1855):221; Annual *Report*, Butler Hospital (1860), excerpted in *AJI* 17 (April 1861):453; Ray, "Examination of the Objections," p. 115; Ray, *Contributions*, pp. 124, 48.

20. O. W. Morris, "An Inquiry whether Deaf Mutes are more Subject to Insanity than the Blind," *AJI* 7 (July 1851):32; Isaac Ray, "Etherization in the Treatment of Insanity," *AJI* 11 (October 1854):185; Ray, *Mental Hygiene*, p. 277; *Report*, State Lunatic Asylum, Jefferson, Mo. (1855), excerpted in *AJI* 12 (April 1856):366.

This period marked the height of the mechanist-vitalist controversy in physiology. See G. June Goodfield, *The Growth of Scientific Physiology: Physiological Method and the Mechanist-Vitalist Controversy* (New York: Arno Press, 1975). Goodfield argues that the debate—whether life processes can be explained strictly in chemical terms or whether some further, "vital," principle is required—was largely a methodological one. Robert Schofield, *Mechanism and Materialism: British Natural Philosophy in an Age of Reason* (Princeton: Princeton University Press, 1970), shows the origins of mechanism and materialism in Newtonian physics.

21. Benedict Morel, *Traité des Dégénérescences Physiques, Intellectualles et Morales de l'Espèce Humanie* (Paris: J. B. Bailliere, 1857), p. 54.

22. See Grob, *The State and the Mentally Ill;* also J. Sanbourne Bockoven, "Moral Treatment in American Psychiatry," *Journal of Nervous and Mental Disease* 74 (August–September 1956), pp. 167-94, 292-321, which deals, in part, with the transition from Ray's generation of asylum superintendents to Gray's; see also J. Sanbourne Bockoven, *The Moral Treatment in American Psychiatry* (New York: Springer, 1963); Eric Carlson and Norman Dain, "The Psychotherapy that was Moral Treatment," *American Journal of Psychiatry* 117 (December 1960):519-24; Ruth Caplan, *Psychiatry and the Community in Nineteenth Century America* (New York: Basic Books, 1969). See Charles Rosenberg's *The Trial of the Assassin Guiteau: Psychiatry and Law in the Gilded Age* (Chicago: University of Chicago Press, 1963), for insight into the later stages of the moral insanity controversy.

23. [John Gray], "Case of Mania with the Delusions and Phenomena of Spiritualism," *AJI* 16 (January 1860):321-40.

24. On the reflex-arc concept, see Edward Liddell, *The Discovery of the Reflexes* (Oxford: Clarendon Press, 1960); F. Fearing, *Reflex Action: A Study in the History of Physiological Psychology* (Baltimore: Williams and Wilkins,

1930); and M. Peter Amacher, "Thomas Laycock, I. N. Sechenov, and the Reflex Arc Concept," *Bulletin of the History of Medicine* 38 (March-April 1964):168-83.

25. John Gray, review of Thomas Henry Buckle's *History of Civilization in England* (1861), in *AJI* 18 (July 1861):70-80; John Gray, "The Study of Mind," *AJI* 17 (January 1861):233-49.

26. See Stow Persons, *The Decline of American Gentility* (New York: Columbia University Press, 1973).

27. Richard Hofstadter, *Anti-Intellectualism in American Life* (New York: Alfred A. Knopf, 1963), p. 106.

28. Persons, *Decline of American Gentility*, pp. 155, 206, 231, 246.

29. S. Weir Mitchell, *Constance Trescot* (New York: The Century Company, 1909), p. 285. For accounts of Mitchell's life and work see: Anna Robeson Burr, *Weir Mitchell: His Life and Letters* (New York: Duffield and Co., 1929); Ernest Earnest, *S. Weir Mitchell, Novelist, and Physician* (Philadelphia: University of Pennsylvania Press, 1950); Joseph Lovering, *S. Weir Mitchell* (New York: Twayne Publishers, 1971); David Rein, *S. Weir Mitchell as a Psychiatric Novelist* (New York: International Universities Press, 1952); Richard Walter, *S. Weir Mitchell, M.D., Neurologist: A Medical Biography* (Springfield, Ill.: Charles C. Thomas, Publisher, 1970).

30. S. Weir Mitchell, *John Sherwood, Ironmaster* (New York: The Century Company, 1914), pp. 210, 241.

31. S. Weir Mitchell, *Dr. North and His Friends* (New York: The Century Company, 1909), p. 389.

32. George Beard, "Neurasthenia or Nervous Exhaustion," *Boston Medical and Surgical Journal* 3 (April 1869):217-21 (hereafter *BMSJ*); idem, "Neurasthenia and its Treatment," *BMSJ* 90 (April 1874):369-70; idem, "The Nature and Diagnosis of Neurasthenia (Nervous Exhaustion)," *The New York Medical Journal* 30 (March 1879):225-51; idem, *A Practical Treatise on Nervous Exhaustion (Neurasthenia): Its Symptoms, Nature, Sequences, Treatment* (New York: William Wood and Company, 1880); idem, *American Nervousness: Its Causes and Consequences* (New York: G. P. Putnam's Sons, 1881). See also, J. L. Teed, "Cerebral Hyperaemia," *The Journal of Nervous and Mental Disease* 4 (April 1877):294 (hereafter *JNMD*); Edward Cowles, *Neurasthenia and Its Symptoms* (Boston: David Clapp, 1891), pp. 21, 10-12; J. S. Jewell, "The Varieties and Causes of Neurasthenia," *JNMD* 7 (January 1880):1-6; Theodore Fisher, "Neurasthenia," *BMSJ* 9 (February 1872):65-72; George Schweig, "Cerebral Exhaustion," *New York Medical Record*, 11 (October 1876):715-17. It was Emil Du Bois-Reymond who, in *Unterschungen über thierische Elektricitat* (Berlin: G. Reimer, 1848), first convincingly claimed to prove the identity of electricity with nerve processes (*Nervenwessens*).

For accounts of Beard see Charles Rosenberg, "The Place of George M. Beard in Nineteenth Century Psychiatry," *Bulletin of the History of Medicine* 36 (May–June 1962):245-59, and the chapter on Beard in his *No Other Gods: On Science and American Thought* (Baltimore: Johns Hopkins Press, 1976), pp. 98-108; M. B. Macmillan, "Beard's Concept of Neurasthenia and Freud's Concept of the Actual Neuroses," *Journal of the History of the Behavioral Sciences* 12 (October 1976):376-90; Henry Alden Bunker, "From Beard to Freud. A Brief History of the Concept of Neurasthenia," *Medical Review of Reviews* 36 (March 1930):109-14; Philip Weiner, "G. M. Beard and Freud on 'American Nervousness,'" *Journal of the History of Ideas* 17 (April 1956):269-74.

33. Fink, *Causes of Crime;* Haller, *Eugenics;* Genil-Perrin, *Dégénérescence en médicine;* Jacques-Joseph Moreau (de Tours), *Du Hachisch et de l'aliénation mentale* (Paris: Fortin, Masson et cie, 1845). See John Hughlings Jackson, "The Factors of Insanity" (1884), in *Selected Writings,* ed. James Taylor, 2 vols. (New York: Basic Books, 1958), 2. Discussions of this movement are incomplete, but see Henri Ellenberger, *The Discovery of the Unconscious* (New York: Basic Books, 1970), pp. 290-91; Franz Alexander and Sheldon Selesnick, *The History of Psychiatry* (New York: Harper and Row, 1966), pp. 159-60; Erwin Stengel, "The Origin and Status of Dynamic Psychiatry," *British Journal of Medicine and Psychiatry* 27, part 41, (1959):193-200; Arthur Lessek, *The Unique Legacy of Doctor Hughlings Jackson* (Springfield, Ill.: Charles C. Thomas, 1970); Owsei Temkin, *The Falling Sickness: A History of Epilepsy from the Greeks to the Beginnings of Modern Neurology* (Baltimore: Johns Hopkins Press, 1945), p. 300. Jackson is discussed in Walter Riese, *A History of Neurology* (New York: MD Publications, 1959), and A. Meyer, *Historical Aspects of Cerebral Anatomy* (London: Oxford University Press, 1971).

34. John Charles Bucknill and Daniel Tuke, *A Manual of Psychological Medicine* (Philadelphia: Blanchard and Lea, 1858), p. 193.

35. "Periscope," *JNMD* 11 (July 1855):537-38.

36. Editorial, *BMSJ* 105 (July 1881):89; "Method in Madness," ibid., pp. 93-95.

37. Edward Spitzka, "Remarkable Automatism in an Epileptic," *New York Medical Record,* 20 (December 1881):733; Edward Spitzka, "The Whitechapel Murders: Their Medical-Legal and Historical Aspects," *JNMD* 15 (December 1888):778; Theodore Fisher, "The Study of Insanity," *BMSJ* 1 (March 1868):66-67; J. S. Wight, "A Plea for the Treatment of Criminals," *American Journal of Neurology and Psychiatry* 3 (May 1884):135-36; James McBride, "The Mental Status of Guiteau—A Review," *Alienist and Neurologist* 4 (October 1883):556; H. Tyler, "A Study of the Laws and Conditions which Govern Human Conduct," *AJI* 48 (April 1892):495; George Beard, "The

Case of Guiteau—a Psychological Study," *JNMD* 9 (January 1882):112.

38. Smith Baker, "Etiological Significance of Heterogeneous Personality," *JNMD* 18 (October 1893):671-72.

39. Edward Cowles, "Neurasthenia and Its Mental Symptoms," *BMSJ* 125 (July 1891):125, 126, 153.

40. Beard, *American Nervousness*, pp. 118, 120, 121.

41. See observations by Rosenberg, "The Place of George M. Beard," pp. 245-59.

42. Edward Spitzka, "Insane Delusions: Their Mechanism and their Diagnostic Bearing," *JNMD* 8 (January 1881):35.

43. James Hendrie Lloyd, "Hysteria: A Study in Psychology," *JNMD* 10 (October 1883):602.

44. J. S. Jewell, "Nervous Exhaustion or Neurasthenia in its Bodily and Mental Relations," *JNMD* 6 (January 1879):53.

45. Bucknill and Tuke, *Manual*, pp. 385-86, 193.

46. Henry Maudsley, *Physiology and Pathology of Mind* (New York: D. Appleton and Company, 1867), p. 159.

47. Beard, *American Nervousness*, p. 97; Nathan Allen, "Physical Degeneracy," *The Journal of Psychological Medicine* 4 (October 1870):756; William Krauss, "The Stigmata of Degeneracy," *AJI* 55 (July 1898):86-87; John Chapin, "The Psychology of Criminals," *AJI* 56 (October 1899):319; T. Edwards Clark, "The Dangerous Classes of the Community," *The Quarterly Journal of Psychological Medicine and Medical Jurisprudence* 1 (October 1867):213.

48. Walter Channing, "Physical Education of Children," *AJI* 48 (January 1892):310; James Kiernan, "Race and Insanity," *JNMD* 13 (July 1886):389-92; Irving Rosse, "Clinical Evidences of Borderline Insanity," *JNMD* 17 (October 1890):669.

49. T. L. Wright, "The Equitable Responsibility of Insanity," *JNMD* 17 (December 1892):871, 873.

50. T. D. Crothers, "Inebriate Automatism," *JNMD* 11 (April 1884):213.

CHAPTER 2. IN SEARCH OF THE REAL MISS BEAUCHAMP

1. Karl Menninger et al., *The Vital Balance: The Life Process in Mental Health and Balance* (New York: Viking Press, 1963), pp. 464-65.

2. Charles Rosenberg, *The Trial of the Assassin Guiteau: Psychiatry and Law in the Gilded Age*, (Chicago: University of Chicago Press, 1963), p. 250.

3. Alfred Binet, *Alterations of Personality*, trans. Helen Green Baldwin (New York: D. Appleton and Co., 1896), p. 235; Henri Ellenberger, *The Discovery of the Unconscious* (New York: Basic Books, 1970), p. 375.

4. Alan Gauld, *The Founders of Psychical Research* (New York: Schocken Books, 1968); Ellenberger, *Discovery of the Unconscious*, ch. 2.

5. Jacques-Joseph Moreau, *Du Hachisch et de l'aliénation mentale* (Paris; Fortin, Masson et cie, 1845), pp. 350-51, 36.

6. Pierre Janet, *The Mental State of Hystericals*, trans. Caroline Corson (New York: G. P. Putnam's Sons, 1901), pp. 354, 250-53, 418, 460.

7. Walter Channing, "The Evolution of Paranoia—Report of a Case," *JNMD* 18 (March 1892):199.

8. William Hammond, "Morbid Impulse," *The Psychological and Medico-Legal Journal* 1 (January 1874):75.

9. James Hendrie Lloyd, "Hysteria," in *A Text-Book on Nervous Diseases by American Authors*, ed. Francis Dercum (Philadelphia: Lea Brothers, 1895), pp. 93, 98, 101, 129.

10. H. M. Bannister, "Emotional Insanity in its Medico-Legal Relations," *JNMD* 7 (January 1880):78-98.

11. T. L. Wright, "Movements of the Human Mind when Placed at a Disadvantage—a Psychological Study," *JNMD* 17 (September 1892):688; Idem, "The Equitable Responsibility of Inebriety," *JNMD* 17 (December 1892):873, 876.

12. Smith Baker, "Etiological Significance of Heterogeneous Personality," *JNMD* 18 (October 1893):671-72.

13. Richard Dewey, "A Case of Disordered Personality," *Journal of Abnormal Psychology* 2 (October-November 1907):141-54.

14. See Putnam's critique of Prince's *The Dissociation of a Personality* in *Journal of Abnormal Psychology*, 1 (October 1906):236-39. For Prince's earliest writing on the subject, see his "Some of the Revelations of Hypnotism, Post Hypnotic Suggestion, Automatic Writing and Double Personality," *BMSJ* 122 (May 1890):463-67, 475-76, 493-95. For a summary of Prince's ideas and his study of Miss Beauchamp, see Nathan Hale, *Freud and the Americans* (New York: Oxford University Press, 1971), pp. 116-32, and his introduction to *Psychotherapy and Multiple Personality: Selected Essays by Morton Prince*, ed. Nathan Hale (Cambridge, Mass.: Harvard University Press, 1975), pp. 1-18; Otto Marx, "Morton Prince and the Dissociation of a Personality," *Journal of the History of the Behavioral Sciences* 6 (April 1970):120-30. Other essays on Prince include: Otto Marx, "Morton Prince and Psychopathology," in *Psychoanalysis, Psychotherapy and the New England Medical Scene*, ed. George Gifford (New York: Science History Publications/U.S.A., 1978), pp. 155-61; Merril Moore, "Morton Prince, M.D. (1854-1929)," *JNMD* 87 (June 1938):701; Henry Murray, "Morton Prince, Sketch of his Life and Work," *Journal of Abnormal and Social Psychology* 52 (May 1956):291-95; William Taylor, *Morton Prince and Abnormal Psychol-*

ogy (New York: D. Appleton and Co., 1928). For the history and criticism of multiple personality theory, see William Taylor and M. F. Martin, "Multiple Personality," *Journal of Abnormal and Social Psychology* 39 (July 1944): 281-300.

15. BCA, "My Life as a Dissociated Personality," *Journal of Abnormal Psychology* for 1908 and 1909, reprinted in Morton Prince, *Clinical and Experimental Studies in Personality* (Cambridge, Mass.: Harvard University Press, 1929), pp. 209-29.

16. Quoted by Morton Prince in *The Unconscious*, 2d rev. ed. (New York: Macmillan Co., 1924), p. 558.

17. Ibid., pp. 567, 579.

18. Ibid., p. 586. See also Morton Prince, "Hysteria from the Point of View of Dissociated Personality," *Journal of Abnormal Psychology* 1 (October 1906):170-87.

19. Prince, *Studies in Personality*, p. viii.

20. "My Life as a Dissociated Personality," p. 221.

21. Ibid., p. 216.

22. Morton Prince, *The Dissociation of a Personality* (London: Longmans, Green and Co., 1920), p. 9.

23. Ibid., pp. 26, 29.

24. Ibid., pp. 53, 86.

25. Ibid., p. 121.

26. Ibid., pp. 111, 106, 138.

27. Ibid., p. 250.

28. Ibid., pp. 185, 186, 236, 213.

29. Ibid., p. 240.

30. Ibid., pp. 463-72.

31. Ibid., pp. 321, 451, 524.

32. Ibid., p. 158.

33. Ibid., pp. 92, 136, 252, 446.

34. Ibid., pp. 493-94.

35. Ibid., pp. 245, 276, 280.

36. Ibid., pp. 266-67, 416, 400-401, 516, 518.

37. Ibid., p. 245.

38. Ibid., p. 517.

39. Sigmund Freud and Joseph Breuer, *Studies in Hysteria*, trans. James Strachey (New York: Basic Books, 1957), p. 287.

40. Ellenberger, *Discovery of the Unconscious*, pp. 539-40.

41. Sigmund Freud, "Notes Upon a Case of Obsessional Neurosis" (1909), *Collected Papers*, 5 vols., trans. James Strachey (New York: Basic Books, 1959), 3:293-384.

42. Ibid., p. 305.

43. Ibid., pp. 313-14.

44. Freud's footnote: "All of this is of course true only in the roughest way, but it serves as a first introduction to the subject." Ibid., p. 315.

45. Ibid., pp. 318, 346, 343.

46. Ibid., pp. 375-76.

47. Ibid., p. 383.

CHAPTER 3. A VOICE FROM THE ABYSS: WILLIAM JAMES

1. The classic study of James, Ralph Barton Perry's *The Thought and Character of William James*, 2 vols. (Boston: Little, Brown and Co., 1935) emphasizes the side of healthy minded moralism. See also, Horace Kallen, "Introduction," *The Philosophy of William James* (New York: Modern Library, 1925); A. J. Ayer, *The Origins of Pragmatism* (San Francisco: Freeman, Cooper, 1968); Edward Moore, *American Pragmatism: Peirce, James and Dewey* (New York: Columbia University Press, 1961); Arthur Bently, "The Jamesian Datum," *Inquiry into Inquiries*, ed. Sidney Ratner (Boston: Beacon Press, 1954); John Smith, "Radical Empiricism," *Proceedings of the Aristotelian Society* 65 (October 1965):205-18; Craig Eisendrath, *The Unifying Moment: The Psychological Philosophies of William James and Alfred North Whitehead* (Cambridge: Harvard University Press, 1971); A. O. Lovejoy, *The Thirteen Pragmatisms and Other Essays* (Baltimore: Johns Hopkins Press, 1963).

For a sick-souled James, see Gay Wilson Allen, *William James: A Biography* (New York: The Viking Press, 1967); Leon Edel, *Henry James, 1870-1881, The Conquest of London* (New York: J. B. Lippincott, 1962); Cushing Strout, "William James and the Twice-Born Sick Soul," *Daedalus* 97 (Summer 1968):1062-82.

More recent works try to strike a balance. See David Marcell, *Progress and Pragmatism: James, Dewey, Beard and the Idea of Progress* (Westport, Conn.: Greenwood Press, 1974); Patrick Dooley, *Pragmatism as Humanism: The Philosophy of William James* (Chicago: Nelson-Hall, 1974); Israel Scheffler, *Four Pragmatists: A Critical Introduction to Peirce, James, Mead, and Dewey* (New York: Humanities Press, 1974); Charlene Seigfried, *Chaos and Context: A Study in William James* (Athens: Ohio University Press, 1978). Also relevant to the present chapter is Thomas Martland's *The Metaphysics of William James and John Dewey; Process and Structure in Philosophy and Religion* (1963; reprint ed., New York: Greenwood Press, 1969).

2. William James (hereafter WJ), to Thomas Ward, December 30, 1876, in Perry, *Thought and Character*, 1:374; WJ to Henry James, Jr., January 22, 1876, in ibid., 1:365; quoted by Allen, *William James*, p. 258.

3. WJ to Thomas Ward, January 1868, in WJ, *The Letters of William James*, 2 vols., ed. Henry James (Boston: Atlantic Monthly Press, 1920), 1:131; WJ to C. Stumpf, May 26, 1893, in Perry, *Thought and Character*, 2:184; WJ to Henry James, Jr., June 12, 1869, William James Papers, Houghton Library, Harvard University, Cambridge, Mass.

4. WJ to Oliver Wendell Holmes, Jr., May 15, 1868, in Perry, *Thought and Character*, 1:514; WJ to Henry James, Jr., October 2, 1869, in ibid., 1:307.

5. WJ to Henry James, Jr., July 15, 1865, Perry, ibid., 1:222; WJ to Henry James, Jr., May 22, 1869, ibid., 1:294.

6. John Jay Chapman, *Memories and Milestones* (Freeport, New York: Books for Libraries Press, 1971), p. 26.

7. WJ, "Diary Note Book, 1868," April 21, 1868, James Papers.

8. WJ, "The Dilemma of Determinism," (1884) in *A William James Reader*, ed. Gay Wilson Allen (Boston: Houghton Mifflin Co., 1971), p. 32.

9. WJ, "Diary Note Book, 1868," May 27, 1868.

10. WJ to Thomas Ward, May 24, 1868, Perry, *Thought and Character*, 1:276; WJ to Alice James, March 16, 1868, ibid., 1:266-67; "Diary Note Book, 1868," December 21, 1868.

11. James was more dogmatic on this point than the physicists themselves, some of whom were wrestling with the questions of models and analogies, others who wished to reduce atomic theory to pure mathematics. See Richard Olson, *Scottish Philosophy and British Physics, 1750-1870* (Princeton: Princeton University Press, 1975); Robert Kargon, "Model and Analogy in Victorian Science," *Journal of the History of Ideas* 30 (July-September 1969):423-36. See Joshua Gregory, *A Short History of Atomism* (London: A. and C. Black, 1931), pp. 81-94, for nineteenth-century skepticism, and W. H. Brock and D. M. Knight, "The Atomic Debates," in *The Atomic Debates*, ed. W. H. Brock, (Leicester: Leicester University Press, 1967), for opposition within chemistry to Dalton's solid, indestructible particle. Wilson Scott, *The Conflict between Atomism and Conservation Theory, 1644-1860* (London: Macdonald and Co., 1970), looks at the opposition to Dalton's hard-body (inelastic) atom and at the compromise elastic molecule with hard-body atoms.

12. See Edward Liddell, *The Discovery of the Reflexes* (Oxford: Clarendon Press, 1960); Peter Amacher, *Freud's Neurological Education and Its Influence on Psychoanalytic Theory*, vol. 4, *Psychological Issues* (New York: International Universities Press, 1965); Robert Young, *Mind, Brain and Adaptation in the Nineteenth Century. Cerebral Localization and its Biological Context from Gall to Ferrier* (Oxford: Clarendon Press, 1970).

13. Perry, *Thought and Character*, 1:520.

14. Quoted in ibid., 1:500.

15. WJ, *The Principles of Psychology,* 2 vols. (1890; reprint ed., New York: Dover Publications, 1950), 1:224, 284, 289.

16. WJ, "Diary Note Book, 1868," February 1, 1870.

17. See John Dewey, "The Vanishing Subject in the Psychology of William James," *Journal of Philosophy* 37 (October 1940):589-99; and the reply by Milic Capek, "The Reappearance of the Self in the Last Philosophy of William James," *Philosophical Review* 57 (October 1953):526-44.

18. WJ, *Principles,* 1:292-301.

19. See Richard Stevens, *James and Husserl: The Foundations of Meaning* (The Hague: Martinus, Nijhoff, 1974), pp. 81-82; Johannes Linschoten, *On the Way Towards a Phenomenological Psychology: The Psychology of William James,* trans. A. Giorgi (Pittsburgh: Duquesne University Press, 1968); John Wild, *The Radical Empiricism of William James,* (Garden City: Doubleday, 1969); Bruce Wilshire, *William James and Phenomenology: A Study of the Principles of Psychology* (Bloomington, Ind.: University of Indiana Press, 1968); James Edie, "Necessary Truth and Perception," in *New Essays in Phenomenology,* ed. James Edie (Chicago: Quadrangle Books, 1965); Robert Elman, "William James and the Structure of the SELF," in ibid. For James's discussion of the passing thought, see *Principles,* 1:344, 340.

20. WJ, *Principles,* 2:125-26.

21. Ibid., 2:540.

22. Noted by Allen, *William James,* p. 164.

23. Henry Maudsley, *Physiology and Pathology of Mind* (New York: D. Appleton and Company, 1867), pp. 144-64.

24. Allen, *William James,* pp. 168-69; Perry, *Thought and Character,* 2:6; Alexander Bain, *The Senses and the Intellect* (London: J. W. Parker and Son, 1855), pp. 61, 54, 327.

25. WJ to Henry James, Jr., October 2, 1869, Perry, *Thought and Character,* 1:306; WJ to Henry Bowditch, December 29, 1869, ibid., 1:320; WJ to Henry James, Jr., May 25, 1873, ibid., 1:346.

26. "Of all departments of medicine, that to which Dr. Prince devotes himself is, I should think, the most interesting. And I should like to see him and his patients at Northampton very much before coming to a decision." WJ to Katharine James Prince, September 12, 1863, *Letters of William James,* 1:44.

27. The date proposed by Allen, *William James,* p. 163.

28. WJ to Henry James, Jr., June 1, 1869 and August 24, 1872, James Papers.

29. WJ, *The Varieties of Religious Experience* (London: Longmans, Green and Co., 1935), p. 160.

30. WJ, "Diary Note Book, 1868," April 30, 1870.

31. WJ, *Varieties*, pp. 162, 163.

32. Ibid., pp. 491-92.

33. Ibid., pp. 161, 151; WJ, *Principles*, 2:298.

34. WJ to George Howison, July 17, 1895, Perry, *Thought and Character*, 2:208; WJ to Thomas Ward, 1869, ibid., 1:160-61; WJ, "Diary Note Book, 1868," April 10, 1873.

35. Henry James, Sr. to Henry James, Jr., 1873, Perry, *Thought and Character*, 1:339-40.

36. Ibid., 1:323.

37. Ibid., 1:521.

38. See Charles Renouvier, *Traité de Psychologie Rationnelle*, vol. 2, *Deuxième Essai* (Paris: A. Colin, 1912), pp. 67-71.

39. Perry, *Thought and Character*, 1:528.

40. This despite the fact that in the *Principles* he continued at times to explain mental illness in terms of the higher-lower doctrine.

41. WJ, *Principles*, 1:72.

42. Ibid., chapter 3.

43. WJ, "What is an Emotion?" (1884), in *Collected Essays and Reviews* (New York: Russell and Russell, 1920), p. 254.

44. WJ, *Principles*, vol. 2, chapter 26.

45. Ibid., 2:197; *Varieties*, p. 499.

46. WJ, *Principles*, 1:173.

47. Particularly, James discovered the famous medium, Mrs. W. J. Piper, in 1885.

48. Perry, *Thought and Character*, 2:156-57.

49. Professor Lightner Witmer held that "William James deliberately opens a campaign for occultisms," and " . . . it is William James *versus* science," in Perry, ibid., 2:153.

50. WJ, *Varieties*, p. 53; *Principles*, 2, Chapter 28.

51. WJ, *Varieties*, p. 7.

CHAPTER 4. COMMUNITY: APOTHEOSIS OF THE REAL MISS BEAUCHAMP

1. William James to Henry Bowditch, July 19, 1880, in Ralph Barton Perry, *The Thought and Character of William James*, 2 vols. (Boston: Little, Brown and Co., 1935), 1:382.

2. G. Stanley Hall, "The Muscular Conception of Space," Mind 3 (October 1878):450; "Psychological Literature," *American Journal of Psychology* 3 (February 1891):578-91, 590.

3. Hall, "The Muscular Conception of Space," p. 446.

4. Hall, "Psychological Literature," p. 590.

5. G. Stanley Hall, *Life and Confessions of a Psychologist* (New York: D. Appleton and Co., 1924), p. 377.

6. Dorothy Ross, *G. Stanley Hall: The Psychologist as Prophet* (Chicago: University of Chicago Press, 1972), p. 11.

7. Hall, *Confessions*, pp. 7, 5.

8. Hall founded and simultaneously edited three journals: *The American Journal of Psychology* (1887); *Pedagogical Seminary* (1891); *The American Journal of Religious Psychology and Education* (1904). Also, he tried in vain to get control of the American wing of the psychoanalytic movement by offering two of its founders, Smith Ely Jelliffe and William Alanson White, the pages of the *American Journal of Psychology* as an alternative to their proposed *Psychoanalytic Review.*

9. G. Stanley Hall, "A Leap Year's Romance," in *Recreations of a Psychologist* (New York: D. Appleton and Co., 1920), p. 261.

10. G. Stanley Hall, "The Education of the Will," *Princeton Review* 10 (November 1882):311, 315, 321.

11. G. Stanley Hall, School Composition #8, 1857, Hall Papers, Clark University.

12. G. Stanley Hall to father, May 13, 1864, Hall Papers.

13. G. Stanley Hall to sister, June 1864, Hall Papers.

14. G. Stanley Hall to parents, 1866, Hall Papers; to mother, January 28, 1866, ibid.; to mother, May 16, 1866, ibid; to mother, February or March 23, 1867, ibid.

15. G. Stanley Hall to mother, February 10, 1869, ibid.

16. G. Stanley Hall, *Adolescence, its Psychology*, 2 vols. (New York: D. Appleton and Co., 1905), 2:45, 292-93.

17. G. Stanley Hall, Miscellaneous speeches, Series IV, Hall Papers.

18. Hall, *Adolescence*, 1:241-42.

19. Ibid., 1:311-12.

20. Ibid., 1:304, 108-12.

21. Ibid., 1:190.

22. Ibid., 2:66.

23. R. Jackson Wilson, *In Quest of Community: Social Philosophy in the United States, 1860-1920* (New York: John Wiley and Sons, Inc., 1968).

24. Hall, *Adolescence*, 1:169, 334; 2:51.

25. Hall, "The Fall of Atlanta," in *Recreations*, pp. 2-127.

26. Hall, *Adolescence*, 1:45.

27. Ibid., 1:444; 2:68.

28. Ibid., 2:124, 123.

29. Ibid., 2:136, 137.

30. Ibid., 2:335.

31. Ibid., 2:544-45.

32. Charles Francis Adams, "Some Phases of Sexual Morality and Church Discipline in Colonial New England," *Proceedings of the Massachusetts Historical Society* 8 (1891):502; John McMasters, *History of the People of the United States*, 6 vols. (New York: D. Appleton and Co., 1885), 2:578-82.

33. For discussions of the early history of the rationalist response to enthusiasm in the Great Awakening see Joseph Haroutunian, *Piety Versus Moralism: The Passing of the New England Theology* (New York: Henry Holt and Co., 1932), and Alan Heimert, *Religion and the American Mind: From the Great Awakening to the Revolution* (Cambridge, Mass.: Harvard University Press, 1966).

34. G. Stanley Hall, "The Moral and Religious Training of Children and Adolescents," *Pedagogical Seminary* 1 (June 1891):191-210.

35. Arthur Daniels, "The New Life: A Study of Regeneration," *American Journal of Psychology* 6 (October 1893):62.

36. Edward Tylor, *Primitive Culture: Researches into the Development of Mythology, Philosophy, Religion, Language, Art and Custom*, 2d. ed. (London: John Murray, 1873), pp. 445, 443-44.

37. Max Müller, *Natural Religion* (London: Longmans, Green and Co., 1889).

38. Tylor, *Primitive Culture*, p. 315; Andrew Lang, *Myths, Ritual and Religion*, 2 vols. (London: Longmans, Green and Co., 1901), 1:57-58.

39. James Leuba, "Professor William James's Interpretation of Religious Experience," *International Journal of Ethics* 14 (April 1904):331, 333.

40. Josiah Morse, "The Pathology of Religions," *American Journal of Religious Psychology and Education* 1 (August 1905):218, 230; James Leuba, "Faith," ibid., 1 (May 1904):82.

41. Edwin Starbuck, "Contributions to the Psychology of Religion," *American Journal of Psychology* 9 (October 1897):70-124.

42. James Bissett Pratt, *The Psychology of Religious Belief* (New York: The Macmillan Co., 1908), pp. ix, 23, 24, 49, 59, 108, 107.

43. Ibid., pp. 192-94.

44. William James, *The Principles of Psychology*, 2 vols. (New York: Dover Publications, 1950), 1:315.

45. George Herbert Mead, *Mind, Self, and Society: From the Standpoint of a Social Behaviorist*, ed. Charles Morris (Chicago: Phoenix Books, 1962), pp. 173-202; see also, Morris's "Introduction," pp. xx-xxvi.

46. The exception was Irving King, who, though from the University of Chicago and a functionalist, reached opposite conclusions. See, King, *The Differentiation of the Religious Consciousness* (New York: Macmillan Co.,

1905), and *The Development of Religion: A Study in Anthropology and Social Psychology* (New York: The Macmillan Co., 1910). An opposite approach growing out of the Chicago School followed John Dewey's skepticism toward English ethnology's primitive man. Dewey argued that the difference in the primitive's perception of the world and the modern lies in his less evolved technological situation. The primitive has not yet made ends of certain means in the way we have; for example, his tools have not yet become objects (alien) to him; being less alienated from his natural environment, he has a different (not worse) perspective on it. Yet Dewey was attracted to the idea that primitive man's consciousness was less evolved than ours; that, for example, he lacked our powers of generalization and abstraction. John Dewey, "Interpretation of Savage Mind," *The Psychological Review* 9 (May 1902):217-30.

47. George Albert Coe, *The Psychology of Religion* (Chicago: University of Chicago Press, 1916), pp. 15-16.

48. Ibid., p. 27.

49. Ibid., pp. 171, 171-72, 208.

50. Ibid., p. 239.

51. Edward Scribner Ames, *The Psychology of Religious Experience* (Boston: Houghton, Mifflin Co., 1910), pp. 335, 333, 359; see also, Ames, "The Genesis of the Group Spirit," *The Psychological Bulletin* 8 (February 15, 1911):53-54.

52. Ibid., p. 26.

53. These were: Edwin Holt, Walter Marvin, William Pepperrell Montagne, Ralph Barton Perry, Walter Pitkin, Edward Spalding.

54. There were, perhaps, also deeper, more personal reasons for Perry's refusal to adopt James's stream as his reality. Perry wrote that "the realist will in any case escape that sense of dissolution and perceptual flux which must haunt the philosopher who identifies exclusively with the passing events of temporal process." *The Present Conflict of Ideals* (New York: Longmans, Green and Co., 1918), p. 372.

55. In an early essay, "Conceptions and Misconceptions of Consciousness," *The Psychological Review* 11 (July-September 1904):282-96, Perry likened private experiencing to a "dream," and to the experiencing of children, "savages," and "abnormal subjects," but attempted to refute the view that there is some kind of supraindividual consciousness located in society.

56. Ralph Barton Perry, "A Realistic Theory of Independence," in *The New Realism: Cooperative Studies in Philosophy.* eds. Perry et al. (New York: The Macmillan Co., 1912), pp. 99-151; Perry, *Present Philosophical Tendencies* (New York: Longmans, Green and Co., 1912), pp. 74, 84, 100, 109, 306-22, 55, 60-61.

57. Edwin Holt, *The Freudian Wish and its Place in Ethics* (New York: Henry Holt and Co., 1915). Perry also embraced behaviorism. See his *Present Conflict of Ideals*, p. 378.

58. Perry, *Present Philosophical Tendencies*, p. 285.

59. Holt, *Freudian Wish*, pp. 47, 3-4.

60. Ibid., pp. 198-99.

61. Edwin Holt, *The Concept of Consciousness* (New York: The Macmillan Co., 1914), pp. 106-8.

62. Ibid., pp. 288, 295.

63. Edwin Holt, *Animal Drive and the Learning Process: An Essay Toward Radical Empiricism* (New York: Henry Holt and Co., 1931), pp. 100, 241.

64. Ibid., p. v. John Burnham writes of the new psychology of the 1920s: "Now there was control through the bureaucratic society in which the inner need, the individual desire, was carefully manipulated and indulged, person by person, so as to prevent the childish, brutal, perverse, or savage in any man's hidden self from disrupting the predictability of civilization." "The New Psychology: From Narcissism to Social Control," *Change and Continuity in Twentieth-Century America: The 1920's*, ed. David Brody, et al. (Columbus: Ohio State University Press, 1968), p. 398.

CHAPTER 5. THE AMERICANIZATION OF FREUDIANISM AND SCHIZOPHRENIA

1. Several leading scholars of Freud's intellectual background barely mention Hughlings Jackson; see, for example, Ernest Jones, *The Life and Work of Sigmund Freud*, 3 vols. (New York: Basic Books, Inc., 1953), 1:214, 215, 356, 368; Sigmund Bernfeld, "Freud's Earliest Theories and the School of Helmholtz," *Psychoanalytic Quarterly* 13 (July 1944):341-62, and "Freud's Scientific Beginnings," *Imago* 4 (1949):3-19; Peter Amacher, Freud's *Neurological Education*, 59; Henri Ellenberger, *Discovery of the Unconscious*, p. 534; Robert Holt, "A Review of Some of Freud's Biological Assumptions and Their Influence on His Theories," in eds. Norman Greenfield and William Lewis, *Psychoanalysis and Current Biological Thought* (Madison: University of Wisconsin Press, 1979), pp. 94-100; Maria Dorer, *Historiche Grundlagen der Psychoanalyse* (Leipzig: F. Meiner, 1932), pp. 15-16. Raymond Fancher, *Psychoanalytic Psychology: The Development of Freud's Thought* (New York: W. W. Norton, 1973), adheres to Amacher's argument that Freud found the Helmholtz school physiology adequate.

In his introduction to his English translation of Freud's *On Aphasia: A Critical Study* (New York: International Universities Press, 1953), and in three articles, "A Re-evaluation of Freud's Book on Aphasia. Its Significance for Psychoanalysis," *International Journal of Psychoanalysis* 35 (Part II, 1954):85; "The Origin and Status of Dynamic Psychiatry," *British Journal of Medical Psychology* 27 (September 1954):193-99; and, "Hughlings Jackson's Influence in Psychiatry," *British Journal of Psychiatry* 109 (May 1963):348-55, Erwin Stengel argued the case for Hughlings Jackson's level theory as being the source of Freud's theory of regression. Frank Sulloway, *Freud, Biologist of the Mind* (New York: Basic Books, Inc., 1979), pp. 270-72, mentions Jackson in this regard, as does Stanley Jackson in "The History of Freud's Concept of Regression," *Journal of the American Psychoanalytic Association* 17 (July 1969):743-83. Ronald Angel, "Jackson, Freud and Sherrington on the Relation of Brain and Mind," *American Journal of Psychiatry* 118 (September 1962):193-97, points out similarities of approach. See also Henry Ey, "Hughlings Jackson's Principles and the Organo-dynamic Concept of Psychiatry," *American Journal of Psychiatry* 118 (February 1962):673-82.

For works describing the causes and nature of Freud's reception in America, see: Nathan Hale's *Freud and the Americans*, and "From Bergasse XIX to Central Park West: The Americanization of Psychoanalysis, 1919-1940," *Journal of the History of the Behavioral Sciences* 14 (October 1978):299-315; John Burnham, *Psychoanalysis and American Medicine, 1894-1918: Medicine, Science, and Culture*, Vol. 5, *Psychological Issues* (New York: International Universities Press, 1969), and "From Avant-Garde to Specialism: Psychoanalysis in America," *Journal of the History of the Behavioral Sciences* 15 (April 1979):128-34.

2. Freud, *On Aphasia*, p. 9.

3. Ibid., pp. 44-51. Meynert's own metaphor was a "mollusca" with tentacles and claws, *Psychiatry*, trans. B. Sachs (New York: G. P. Putnam's Sons, 1885), 1:139.

4. Freud, *On Aphasia*, 61, 87. See John Hughlings Jackson, "On Affections of Speech from Disease in the Brain," *Selected Writings*, II, 155-204. Since this is the only Jacksonian work Freud cited, I will restrict my discussion to its contents.

5. Joseph Breuer (with Sigmund Freud), *Studies on Hysteria* (1893), *The Standard Edition of the Complete Psychological Works of Sigmund Freud*, 23 vols., ed. James Strachey, (London: The Hogarth Press, 1953-1966), 2:113; Theodor Meynert, *Sammelung von popularwissenschaftlichen Vortragen über den Bau und die Leistungen des Gehirns* (Vienna: W. Braumuller, 1892), p. 12.

6. See my "Sigmund Freud, John H. Jackson, and Speech," to appear in the *Journal of the History of Ideas*.

7. Theodor Meynert, *Psychiatry*, 1:154-59, 167-72.

8. Sigmund Freud, "Project for a Scientific Psychology" (1895), in *The Origins of Psycho-Analysis. Letters to Wilhelm Fliess, Drafts and Notes: 1887-1902*, eds. Marie Bonaparte, Anna Freud, Ernst Kris, trans. Eric Mosbacher, James Strachey (New York: Basic Books, Inc., 1954), p. 386; Sigmund Freud, "A Note on the Unconscious in Psycho-Analysis" (1912), *Collected Papers*, 5 vols., ed. Alix and James Strachey 5 vols. (New York: Basic Books, Inc., 1956), 4:25, 24.

9. Freud, "Project," pp. 357, 359, 384-86, 407; Sigmund Freud, *The Interpretation of Dreams* (1900), *Standard Edition*, 5:597-98.

10. Freud, "Case of Obsessional Neurosis," *Collected Papers*, 3:382-83.

11. Freud, "Project," p. 410.

12. Freud, *Interpretation of Dreams*, 4:160, 78, 5:526, 578-80.

13. Ibid., 4:219, 58, 5:591; Sigmund Freud, *On Dreams* (1901), *Standard Edition*, 5:659-65.

14. Sigmund Freud, *New Introductory Lectures on Psycho-Analysis* (1933), *Standard Edition*, 22:103-4.

15. Smith Ely Jelliffe and William Alanson White, *Diseases of the Nervous System: A Text-Book of Neurology and Psychiatry* (Philadelphia: Lea and Febiger, 1915), p. 682.

16. Ibid., p. 685.

17. Carl Jung, *Psychology of Dementia Praecox*, trans. Frederick Peterson and A. A. Brill (New York: The Journal of Nervous and Mental Disease Publishing Co., 1909), p. 36.

18. Eugene Bleuler, *Dementia Praecox, or, The Group of Schizophrenias*, trans. Joseph Zinker (New York: International Universities Press, 1950), p. 29.

19. Jelliffe and White, *Diseases of the Nervous System*, p. 687. This in stark contrast with White's pre-Freudian assertion, is reminiscent of Ray, concerning impulsive acts: "It is quite impossible to get any adequate information as to the cause of these acts.... These acts come out of clear sky, cannot be foreseen, and make these [dementia praecox] patients at times very dangerous." Isaac Ray, *Outlines of Psychiatry* (New York: Nervous and Mental Disease Publishing Company, 1907), p. 156.

20. In one of his rare discussions of schizophrenia, "Psycho-Analytic Notes on an Autobiographical Account of a Case of Paranoia (Dementia Paranoides)" (1911), *Standard Edition*, 12:9-82, Freud attributed the illness to total withdrawal of libido from the object world and its narcissistic attachment to self at the fully regressed state of infantile auto-eroticism. Repression wins its battle, causing failure of the ego. It is the failure of the ego, he said, that distinguishes the psychoses from a mere neurosis like simple paranoia in which libido, though at first withdrawn from the object world and homosexually invested in the self is reprojected in distorted form onto the object world. In the latter case some reality-testing is maintained, but the schizophrenic is

locked into his own fantasy formation and is beyond psychoanalytic help. Freud dealt again with the psychoses, "amentia" and "schizophrenia," in his "A Metaphysical Supplement to the Theory of Dreams" (1917 [1915]), *Standard Edition*, 14:222-35. Here the dream and dream-work become models for the psychoses and their mechanisms. Here he argued that schizophrenia, in contrast to dreaming, involves no topographical regression, because in schizophrenia, as opposed to the dream, the words themselves (system *Cs.*) are worked on and modified by the primary process.

21. John Burnham, *Psychoanalysis and American Medicine, 1894-1918: Medicine, Science, and Culture* (New York: International Universities Press, 1967), p. 138.

22. William Alanson White to G. Stanley Hall, February 11, 1913, Hall Papers, Clark University.

23. Arcangelo D'Amore, "William Alanson White—Pioneer Psychoanalyst," in *William Alanson White: The Washington Years, 1903-1937*, ed. Arcangelo D'Amore (Washington: U.S. Department of Health, Education and Welfare, n.d.), pp. 70-71.

24. Lawrence Moore, "William Alanson White—A Biography (1870-1937)," in ibid., p. 15.

25. Book Review, *JNMD* 62 (September 1925):331; Book Review, ibid., 54 (September 1921):286; Obituary, Sir David Ferrier, ibid. 67 (September 1928):642.

26. S. C. Burchell, "The Frail Sister Forgets Herself," ibid. 68 (September 1928):228.

27. See White's discussion, "The Unconscious," *Psychoanalytic Review* 3 (January 1915):23. Hereafter, *Psa Review.*

28. Walter Cannon, "New Evidence for Sympathetic Control of Some Internal Secretions," *American Journal of Psychiatry* 79 (July 1922):26.

29. James Jackson Putnam, "Sketch for a Study of New England Character" (1917), in *Addresses on Psycho-Analysis* (London: The Hogarth Press, Ltd., 1951), pp. 366-96. See Nathan Hale's essay on Putnam in *James Jackson Putnam and Psychoanalysis: Letters Between Putnam and Sigmund Freud, Ernest Jones, William James, Sandor Ferenczi, and Morton Prince, 1877-1917* (Cambridge: Harvard University Press, 1971); Hale, *Freud and the Americans,* p. 133; Edward Taylor, "James Jackson Putnam: His Contributions to Neurology," *Archives of Neurology and Psychiatry* 3 (March 1920):307-15.

30. James Jackson Putnam, "The Work of Sigmund Freud" (1917), *Addresses*, p. 351.

31. James Jackson Putnam, "The Present State of Psychoanalysis" (1914), *Addresses*, p. 255; ibid., "The Necessity of Metaphysics," p. 307, 310-11; ibid., "Personal Experience with Freud's Psychoanalytic Method," p. 46; ibid., "Sketch for a Study of New England Character," p. 367.

32. Smith Ely Jelliffe and Louise Brink, *Psychoanalysis and the Drama* (Washington: Nervous and Mental Disease Publishing Co., 1922), pp. 2, 9.

33. Smith Ely Jelliffe, *The Technique of Psychoanalysis*, (New York: Nervous and Mental Disease Publishing Co., 1918), p. 66.

34. William Alanson White, "Moon Myth and Medicine," *Psa Review* 1 (July 1914):245.

35. Adolf Meyer, "What is the Safest Psychology for a Nurse?" (1916), *Collected Papers*, 4 vols., ed. Eunice Winters (Baltimore: Johns Hopkins Press, 1950-1952), 4:84; "Mental and Moral Health in a Constructive School Program" (1925), ibid., 4:335.

36. Adolf Meyer, "Remarks on Habit Disorganization in the Essential Deteriorations" (1905), ibid., 2:428: Meyer spoke of "the contemporaneous humanization not only of psychology but of philosophy through William James's espousal of the characteristically American concepts of pragmatism, instrumentalism, and the humanization of religious experience," in "Organization of the Community Facilities for Prevention, Care, and Treatment of Nervous and Mental Diseases" (1930), ibid., 2:271; see also, "The Scientific Study of Behavior and Its Support" (1926), ibid., 2:132; and, "National Conference on Family Relations" (1940), ibid., 2:501. See Frederick Woodbridge, "The Nature of Consciousness," *Journal of Philosophy, Psychology and Scientific Methods* 2 (March 2 1905):119-25 for a statement of his New Realist faith.

37. See, Hale, *Freud and the Americans*, pp. 157-64; Burnham, *Psychoanalysis and American Medicine*, pp. 85-89, 158-61; Eunice Winters, "Adolf Meyer's Two and a Half Years at Kankakee, May 1, 1893-November 1, 1895," *Bulletin of the History of Medicine* 40 (September–October 1966): 441-58; Alfred Lief, *The Commonsense Psychiatry of Dr. Adolf Meyer* (New York: McGraw Hill Publishing Co., 1948).

38. Adolf Meyer, "What Do Histories of Cases of Insanity Teach us Concerning Preventive Hygiene During the Years of School Life?" (1908-1909), *Collected Papers*, 4:346.

39. Adolf Meyer, "Individualism and the Organization of Neuropsychiatric Work in a Community" (1918), ibid., 4:260.

40. Adolf Meyer, "Misconceptions at the Bottom of 'Hopelessness of All Psychology,' " (1907), ibid., 2:580, 579, 576. Information about Meyer's early intellectual career is scattered through his works, in particular his "British Influence in Psychiatry, and Mental Hygiene" (1933), ibid., 3:400-28; see also Lief's interviews with Meyer in *The Commonsense Psychiatry*, and Winters, "Adolf Meyer's Two and a Half Years at Kankakee."

41. Adolf Meyer, "Segmental-Suprasegmental Concept: Critical Review of the Data and General Methods of Modern Neurology" (1898), *Collected Papers*, 1:127, 132; "The Relation of Emotional and Intellectual Functions in

Paranoia and Obsessions" (1906), ibid., 2:500; "Aphasias" (1903), ibid., 1:334-47; "Revision of Aphasia" (1907), ibid., 1:347-68.

42. Ibid., 1:353.

43. William Alanson White to Adolf Meyer, January 5, 1920, Meyer Papers, Johns Hopkins University; William Alanson White, "Critical Review: The Autonomic Functions and the Personality, by Edward J. Kempf," *Psa Review* 6 (January 1919):89-98. In subsequent editions of *Outlines of Psychiatry,* White continued to rank Kempf with Jung, Freud, and Adler, but in 1924 White declined to write an article about Kempf for the *New Republic* on the grounds that Kempf was not important enough. White to *New Republic,* January 18, 1924, White Papers, National Archives. Part of the trouble may be explainable by a letter White received accusing Kempf of stealing White's theoretical thunder. E. H. Reede to White, December 20, 1920, ibid.

44. Edward Kempf, "The Social and Sexual Behavior of Infra-Human Primates with Some Comparable Facts in Human Behavior," *Psa Review* 4 (April 1917):133; *The Autonomic Functions of the Nervous System* (Washington, D.C.: Nervous and Mental Disease Publishing Co., 1918), p. 23. It is possible that Kempf was building on Meyer. In his "The Relation of Emotional and Intellectual Functions in Paranoia and Obsessions," p. 499, Meyer argued: "Broadly speaking, almost every mental activity allows us to recognize relations to two fundamental systems, that of the shaping of the personal physiopsychological ("emotional") attitudes in our circulatory, respiratory and vegetative side, and that of the more fleeting and more impersonal neuromuscular ("intellectual") relations, based on the sense organs *per se* and the muscular apparatus carrying and directing them."

45. Kempf, *Autonomic Functions,* pp. 127, ix, 32-41, 78.

46. Edward Kempf, "The Integrative Functions of the Nervous System Applied to Some Reactions in Human Behavior and their Attending Psychic Functions," *Psa Review* 2 (April 1915):153-55; "Some Studies in the Psychopathology of Acute Dissociation of the Personality," ibid., 2 (October 1915):381-86; *Autonomic Functions,* pp. xiii, 1-3.

47. Kempf, ibid., pp. 95-97, 100, 110.

48. William Alanson White, "The Mechanism of Transference," *Psa Review* 4 (October 1917):273-81.

49. White, "The Unconscious," pp. 22-23.

50. Ibid., pp. 24, 27.

51. See William Alanson White, "The Significance for Psychopathology of Child's Developmental Gradients and the Dynamic Differentiation of the Head Region," *Psa Review* 4 (January 1918):93-103.

52. Charles Child, *Physiological Foundations of Behavior* (New York: Hefner Publishing Co., 1924), pp. 35, 186, 195.

53. White, "Child's Developmental Gradients," pp. 98, 91, 103.

54. William Alanson White, "Extending the Field of Conscious Control," *Psa Review* 7 (April 1920):156. For an outstanding discussion of where the question of emergence and reductionism now stands, see Ernan McMullan, "What Difference Does Mind Make?" *Brain and Human Behavior*, eds. A. G. Karczmar and J. C. Eccles (New York: Springer-Verlag, 1972), pp. 423-47.

55. William Alanson White, "The Unity of the Organism," *Psa Review* 7 (January 1920):77.

56. Adolf Meyer to William Alanson White, October 29, 1919; White to Meyer, November 5, 1919, White Papers.

57. William Alanson White, "Symbolism," *Psa Review* 3 (January 1916):12.

58. Ellenberger, *Discovery of the Unconscious*, p. 236.

59. See chapter 7, but see also C. Judson Herrick's statement in his *The Evolution of Human Nature* (Austin: University of Texas Press, 1956), pp. 311-12; see also Burnham's remarks, *Psychoanalysis and American Medicine*, p. 55.

60. William Alanson White, "The Language of Schizophrenia," in Association for Research in Nervous and Mental Disease, *Schizophrenia (Dementia Praecox) Proceedings* (New York: Paul B. Hoeber, 1928), pp. 323, 333, 334-35.

61. William Alanson White, "Some Considerations Bearing on the Diagnosis and Treatment of Dementia Praecox," *Psa Review* 8 (October 1921):418.

62. Albert Storch, *The Primitive Archaic Forms of Inner Experience and Thought in Schizophrenia*, trans. Clara Willard (New York: Nervous and Mental Disease Publishing Co., 1924), pp. ix, 4, 11.

63. William Alanson White, "The Comparative Method in Psychiatry," *JNMD* 61 (January 1925):14.

64. For the impact of the White circle on psychosomatic medicine, see Robert Powell, "Helen Flanders Dunbar (1902-1959) and a Holistic Approach to Psychosomatic Problems. I. The Rise and Fall of a Medical Philosophy," *Psychiatric Quarterly* 49 (Summer 1977):133-52. The impact of individuals within the circle is discussed in Hale, *Freud in America*, and by Jean Jones, "William Alanson White—Patron of Mental Health," in *William Alanson White*, ed., Arcangelo D'Amore pp. 103-11; and Robert Kvarnes, "The Founding of the William Alanson White Psychiatric Foundation," in ibid., pp. 123-29.

65. See discussions by Roy Lubove, *The Professional Altruist: The Emergence of Social Work as a Career, 1880-1930* (Cambridge: Harvard University Press, 1965), and by John Burnham, "The New Psychology: From Narcissism to Social Control," in *Change and Continuity in Twentieth Century America: The 1920's*, ed. John Braeman et al. (Columbus: Ohio State University Press, 1968), pp. 351-98.

CHAPTER 6. PSYCHIATRY: A FADING SCIENCE

1. H. S. Sullivan, *Conceptions of Modern Psychiatry*, in *Collected Works*, 2 vols., eds. Helen Swick Perry and Mary Ladd Gawel (New York: W. W. Norton, 1954), 1:9.

2. Helen Swick Perry, "Introduction," in H. W. Sullivan, *Schizophrenia as a Human Process* (New York: W. W. Norton, 1962), p. xii. However, another biographer, A. H. Chapman, in his *Harry Stack Sullivan. His Life and Work* (New York: Putnams, 1976), pp. 22-23, has argued that from age eight to ten Sullivan carried on a homosexual relation with a neighbor five years his elder.

3. Clara Thompson, "Harry Stack Sullivan, the Man," in Sullivan, *Schizophrenia as a Human Process*, pp. xxxii-xxv.

4. H. S. Sullivan, *Personal Psychopathology* (New York: W. W. Norton, 1972), p. 180.

5. H. S. Sullivan, "Schizophrenia: Its Conservative and Malignant Features," *American Journal of Psychiatry* 81 (July 1924):77-91.

6. Ibid., p. 83.

7. Helen Swick Perry, "Introduction," in Sullivan, *Personal Psychopathology*, p. xxiii.

8. W. A. White to Ross McC. Chapman, November 21, 1922. White Papers, National Archives.

9. W. A. White to Thomas Haines, Director, Division of Mental Deficiency, National Committee of Mental Hygiene, March 20, 1924. Ibid.

10. Edward Sapir, "Cultural Anthropology and Psychiatry," *Journal of Abnormal and Social Psychology* 27 (October-December 1932):229-42. Sullivan spoke of the "mésalliance of neurology and psychiatry" in his "Conceptions of Modern Psychiatry: The First William Alanson White Memorial Lectures," *Psychiatry* 3 (February 1940):3.

11. W. A. White, "Psychiatry and the Social Sciences," August 1928. White Papers.

12. H. S. Sullivan to W. A. White, August 10, 1929. Sullivan Papers, William Alanson White Institute, Washington, D.C. White to Sullivan, August 12, 1929. Ibid.

13. W. A. White to H. S. Sullivan, September 3, 1929. Ibid.

14. H. S. Sullivan to W. A. White, April 13, 1930. White Papers; Sullivan to White, April 2, 1930. Ibid.; Sullivan to White, April 30, 1930. Sullivan Papers.

15. H. S. Sullivan to W. A. White, May 17, 1930. Sullivan Papers.

16. H. S. Sullivan to W. A. White, May 14, 1930. White Papers.

17. H. S. Sullivan to W. A. White, May 21, 1930. Ibid.

18. H. S. Sullivan to W. A. White, Ibid.; White to Sullivan, June 17, 1930. Ibid.; Sullivan to White, July 5, 1930. Ibid.

19. Franklin Ebaugh, "The Crisis in Psychiatric Education," *Journal of the*

American Medical Association 99 (August 27, 1932):703-6.

20. Franklin Ebaugh to W. A. White, May 14, 1931, White Papers; White to Ebaugh, May 18, 1931. Ibid.

21. W. A. White to H. S. Sullivan, October 25, 1935, Sullivan Papers.

22. Sullivan, "Schizophrenia," p. 90.

23. H. S. Sullivan, "The Oral Complex," *Psa Review* 12 (January 1925):30-38.

24. Sapir, "Cultural Anthropology," pp. 229-42.

25. Edward Sapir, *Language: An Introduction to the Study of Speech* (New York: Harcourt, Brace and Co., 1921), p. 22.

26. H. S. Sullivan, *The Interpersonal Theory of Psychiatry*, eds. Helen Swick Perry and Mary Ladd Gawel (New York: W. W. Norton, 1953), p. 240.

27. Published in installments in *Psychiatry*, and again posthumously in book form *Conceptions of Modern Psychiatry* (New York: W. W. Norton, 1953).

28. Sullivan, *Interpersonal Theory*, pp. 192-202.

29. Ibid., pp. 160-65, 326-27.

30. Ibid., p. 342.

31. Ibid., p. 340.

32. Robert Knight, "Introduction," *Psychotherapy with Schizophrenics*, eds. Eugene Brody and Frederick Redlich (New York: International Universities Press, 1952), p. 4.

33. Norman Cameron, *Personality Development and Psychopathology* (Boston: Houghton, Mifflin Co., 1963), p. 609.

34. C. Peter Rosenbaum, *Meaning of Madness: Symptomatology, Sociology, Biology, and Therapy of the Schizophrenias* (New York: Science House, 1970), p. 236; Silvano Arieti, "The Psychotherapy of Schizophrenia in Theory and Practice," *Psychotherapy of Schizophrenia and Manic-Depressive States*, Psychiatric Research Report 17, eds. Hassan Azima and Bernard Glueck (Washington D.C.: American Psychiatric Association, 1963), p. 14.

35. Sigmund Freud, *Three Essays on the Theory of Sexuality* (1905). *The Standard Edition of the Complete Psychological Works of Sigmund Freud*, 23 vols., ed. James Strachey (London: The Hogarth Press, 1953-66), 7:125.

36. Karl Abraham, "Short Study of the Development of the Libido Viewed in the Light of Mental Disorders" (1924), in *Selected Papers of Karl Abraham*, 2 vols., ed., Ernest Jones, trans. Douglas Bryan and Alix Strachey (London: Basic Books, 1927), 1:418-501.

37. W. R. D. Fairbairn, "A Revised Psychopathology of the Psychoses and Psychoneuroses," *International Journal of Psycho-Analysis* 22 (Parts 3 and 4, 1941):250-79.

38. Ibid., p. 261.

39. Elvin Semrad, "Long-Term Therapy in Schizophrenia," in *Psychoneurosis and Schizophrenia*, ed. Gene Usdin (Philadelphia: J. B. Lippincott, 1966), pp. 160-61.

40. Quoted in *Psychotherapy of Chronic Schizophrenic Patients: Sea Island Conference*, ed. Carl Whitaker (Boston: Little, Brown and Co., 1948), p. 159.

41. Louis Hill, *Psychotherapeutic Intervention in Schizophrenia* (Chicago: University of Chicago Press, 1955), p. 183.

42. Semrad, "Long-Term Therapy," p. 158.

43. Hill, *Psychotherapeutic Intervention*, pp. 183, 140.

44. Leon Saul, *Technic and Practice of Psychoanalysis* (Philadelphia: J. B. Lippincott, 1958), p. 26.

45. Silvano Arieti, "Introductory Notes on the Psychoanalytic Therapy of Schizophrenics," *Psychotherapy of the Psychoses*, ed. Arthur Burton (New York: Basic Books, 1961), p. 78.

46. Carl Whitaker and Thomas Malone, *The Roots of Psychotherapy* (New York: Blakiston, 1953).

47. Julius Steinfeld, *A New Approach to Schizophrenia* (New York: Merlin Press, 1956), pp. 40-43, 57.

48. John Rosen, *Direct Analysis: Selected Papers*, 2 vols. (New York: Grune and Stratton, 1953), 1:8.

49. Quoted in Whitaker, *Sea Island Conference*, p. 114.

50. Quoted in ibid., 80-83.

51. For example, Hill, *Psychotherapeutic Intervention*, 183; Richard Chessick, *How Psychotherapy Heals: The Process of Intensive Psychotherapy* (New York: Science House, 1969), 49; Paul DeWald, *Psychotherapy*, 2nd ed. (Oxford: Blackwell Science Publications, 1969), 215-16.

52. Frieda Fromm-Reichmann, "Transference Problems in Schizophrenia" (1939), *Psychoanalysis and Psychotherapy: Selected Papers of Frieda Fromm-Reichmann*, ed. Dexter Bullard, (Chicago: University of Chicago Press, 1959), p. 125.

53. Hill, *Psychotherapeutic Intervention*, p. 177.

54. Donald Burnham, Arthur Gladstone, and Robert Gibson, *Schizophrenia and the Need-Fear Dilemma* (New York: International Universities Press, 1969), p. 286.

55. William Pious, "A Hypothesis about the Nature of Schizophrenic Behavior," in ed. Arthur Burton, *Psychotherapy of the Psychoses* (New York: Basic Books, 1961), p. 51.

56. But in 1962 A. Rechtshaffen, D. R. Goodenough and A. Shapiro tested this theory in "Patterns of Sleep-Talking," *Archives of General Psychiatry* 12 (December 1962):418-26, and found that sleep-talkers normally

and comprehensively speak in relation to their dreams or the experimental situation.

57. Hans Oppenheimer, *Clinical Psychiatry: Issues and Challenges* (New York: Harper and Row, 1971), pp. 240-42.

58. Leopold Bellak, "The Schizophrenic Syndrome," *Schizophrenia: A Review of the Syndrome,* ed. Leopold Bellak, (New York: Logos Press, 1959), p. 18; Normal Cameron, "Deterioration and Regression in Schizophrenic Thinking," *Journal of Abnormal and Social Psychology* 34 (April 1939):265-70.

59. Otto Allen Will, "The Conditions of Being Therapeutic," *Psychotherapy of Schizophrenia,* eds. John Gunderson and Loren Mosher (New York: Jason Aranson, 1975), pp. 59-63.

60. Margaret Mahler, "On Child Psychosis and Schizophrenia," *The Psychoanalytic Study of the Child* 7 (1952):298.

61. Steinfeld, *New Approach*, pp. 57, 77.

62. Roy Grinker, *Psychosomatic Medicine* (New York: W. W. Norton, 1953), p. 135.

63. Burnham et al., *Schizophrenia and the Need-Fear Dilemma*, p. 33.

64. Chessick, *How Psychotherapy Heals*, pp. 46-47.

65. Charles Savage, "Countertransference in the Theory of Schizophrenia," *Psychiatry* 24 (February 1961):58.

66. Quoted in *Sea Island Conference*, p. 79.

67. Milton Wexler, "The Structural Problem in Schizophrenia," in eds., Eugene Brody and Frederick Redlich *Psychotherapy with Schizophrenics* (New York: International Universities Press, 1952), p. 199.

68. Burnham, *Schizophrenia and the Need-Fear Dilemma*, p. 298.

69. Harold Searles, *The Nonhuman Environment: In Normal Development and in Schizophrenia,* 2d ed. (New York: International Universities Press, 1960), p. 371.

70. Carl Whitaker, "The Commitment to Intimacy," *The Analytic Situation,* ed. Hendrick Ruitenbeek (Chicago: Aldine Publishing Co., 1973), p. 183.

71. Burnham et al., *Schizophrenia and the Need-Fear Dilemma*, p. 291.

72. Jurgen Ruesch, *Disturbed Communication* (New York: W. W. Norton, 1957), pp. 130-31.

73. Otto Allen Will, "Schizophrenia, the Problem of Origins," in *The Origins of Schizophrenia: Proceedings of the First Rochester International Conference on Schizophrenia,* ed. John Romano (Amsterdam, Excerpta Medica Foundation, 1967), p. 223.

74. Savage, "Countertransference," pp. 53-60; Mabel Cohen, "Countertransference and Anxiety," *Psychiatry* 15 (August 1952):231-43.

75. Searles, *Nonhuman Environment*, p. 366.

76. Savage, "Countertransference," p. 58.

77. Fromm-Reichmann, "Remarks on the Philosophy of Mental Disorder" (1949), *Selected Papers*, pp. 3–24.

78. David Wright, "Discussion of Dr. Fromm-Reichmann's Paper," in eds., Brody and Redlich *Psychotherapy and Schizophrenia*, p. 129.

79. Eugene Brody, "The Treatment of Schizophrenia: A Review," in ibid., 44.

80. Hill, *Psychotherapeutic Intervention*, p. 33.

81. Ibid., 193.

82. Savage, "Countertransference," p. 57.

83. Chessick, *How Psychotherapy Heals*, pp. 42, 97.

84. Ibid., p. 97.

85. Harold Searles, "Data Concerning Certain Manifestations of Incorporation" (1951), in Searles, *Collected Papers on Schizophrenia and Related Subjects* (New York: International Universities Press, 1965), p. 63.

86. Robert Knight, "Preface," in Searles, *Collected Papers*, p. 15.

87. Searles, *Nonhuman Environment*, pp. 239, 268, 294.

88. Searles, "Data Concerning Certain Manifestations," pp. 39–69, 68.

89. The idea that deviance is functional to the social process goes back to Emil Durkheim's *The Rules of Sociological Method*, trans. S. A. Solovay and J. H. Mueller (Glencoe, Ill: The Free Press, 1958). My point that the definition of schizophrenia derives from the attempt to save a conceptual mapping may very well be an expression of this general approach. For expressions of the theory that social groups create deviance by making the rules whose infraction constitutes deviance and by applying those rules to particular people, see Frank Tannenbaum, *Crime and the Community* (New York: McGraw-Hill Book Co., Inc., 1951); E. M. Lemert, *Social Pathology* (McGraw-Hill Book Co., Inc., 1951); John Kitsuse, "Societal Reaction to Deviance: Problems of Theory and Method," *Social Problems* 9 (Winter 1962):247-56. For a historical application of this principle, see Kai Erickson, *Wayward Puritans: A Study in the Sociology of Deviance* (New York and London: John Wiley and Sons, 1966).

CHAPTER 7. PSYCHOSURGERY: SCIENCE CONFRONTS THE BIZARRE

1. Eugene Bleuler, *Dementia Praecox, or, The Group of Schizophrenias*, trans. Joseph Zinkin (New York: International Universities Press, 1950), pp. 9, 315.

2. C. Macfie Campbell, *Destiny and Disease in Mental Disorders: With*

Special Reference to Schizophrenic Psychoses (New York: W. W. Norton, 1935), p. 61.

3. J. M. Nielsen and George Thompson, *The Engrammes of Psychiatry* (Springfield, Ill.: Charles C. Thomas, 1947), p. 219.

4. American Psychiatric Association, *Diagnostic and Statistical Manual—Mental Disorders*, 2d ed. (Washington, D.C.: American Psychiatric Association, 1968), p. 33.

5. A. A. Brill, "Psychological Factors in Dementia Praecox," *Journal of Abnormal Psychology* 3 (October–November, 1908):233.

6. Oswald Boltz, "Some Factors which Determine a Schizophrenic (Dementia Praecox) Reaction in Males," *JNMD* 64 (November 1926):459.

7. Karl Jaspers, *General Psychopathology*, trans. J. Hoenig and Marion Hamilton (Chicago: University of Chicago Press, 1963), p. 447.

8. Adolf Meyer, "Nature and Conception of Dementia Praecox" (1910), *Collected Papers*, ed. Eunice Winters, 4 vols. (Baltimore: Johns Hopkins Press, 1950-52), 2:461.

9. Phyllis Greenacre, "The Content of the Schizophrenic Characteristics Occurring in Affective Disorders," *American Journal of Psychiatry* 75 (October 1918):197.

10. William Alanson White, "Primitive Mentality and the Racial Unconscious," *American Journal of Psychiatry* 81 (April 1925):669.

11. William Alanson White, "Some Considerations Bearing on the Diagnosis and Treatment of Dementia Praecox," *American Journal of Psychiatry* 78 (October 1921):144.

12. Boltz, "Some Factors," pp. 459, 463.

13. Jaspers, *General Psychopathology*, p. 447.

14. C. Peter Rosenbaum, *Meaning of Madness, Symptomatology, Sociology, Biology and Therapy of the Schizophrenias* (New York: Science House, 1970), p. 85.

15. E. E. Southard, "The Empathic Index in the Diagnosis of Mental Diseases," *Journal of Abnormal Psychology* 13 (October 1918):211.

16. Nielsen and Thompson, *Engrammes of Psychiatry*, p. 220.

17. American Psychiatric Association, *Diagnostic and Statistical Manual*, 33.

18. Bleuler, *Dementia Praecox, or, The Group of Schizophrenias*, p. 322.

19. Carl Jung, *The Psychology of Dementia Praecox*, trans. Frederick Peterson and A. A. Brill (New York: The Journal of Nervous and Mental Disease Publishing Co., 1909), 74.

20. White, "Some Considerations," pp. 193-98, 197.

21. Robert Gibson, "The Ego Defect in Schizophrenia," *Psychoneurosis and Schizophrenia*, ed. Gene Usdin (Philadelphia: J. B. Lippincott Co., 1966), p. 91.

22. Walter Freeman and James Watts, *Psychosurgery: In the Treatment of Mental Disorders and Intractable Pain*, 2d ed. rev. (Springfield, Ill.: Charles C. Thomas, 1950), pp. 299, 524.

23. R. S. Woodworth and C. S. Sherrington, "A Pseudoaffective Reflex and its Spinal Path," *Journal of Physiology* 31 (June 30, 1904):234-43.

24. Henry Head and Gordon Holmes, "Sensory Disturbances for Cerebral Lesions," *Brain* 34 (Pts. 3, 4, 1911-12):102-254.

25. Walter Cannon, "New Evidence for Sympathetic Control of Some Internal Secretions," *American Journal of Psychiatry* 79 (July 1922):15-30; Cannon and S. W. Britton, "Studies on the Conditions of Activity in Endocrine Glands," *American Journal of Physiology* 72 (April 1, 1925):283-94; Cannon, "The James-Lange Theory of Emotions: A Critical Examination and an Alternative Theory," *American Journal of Psychology* 39 (December 1927):106-24; Philip Bard, "A Diencephalic Mechanism for the Expression of Rage, with Special Reference to the Sympathetic Nervous System," *American Journal of Physiology* 84 (April 1, 1928):490-515; Bard, "On Emotional Expression after Decortication with some Remarks on Certain Theoretical Views," *Psychological Review* 41 (July 1934):309-29.

26. Recent experiments have supported James on this point. See, Steward Wolf and Harold Wolff, *Human Gastric Function*, 2d ed. (New York: Oxford University Press, 1947); Albert Ax, "The Physiological Differentiation between Fear and Anger," *Psychosomatic Medicine* 15 (September-October 1953): 433-42; Joseph Schlachter, "Pain, Fear, and Anger in Hypersensitives and Normotensives," ibid. 19 (January-February 1957):17-29; Francis Graham and Nancy Kunish, "Physiological Responses of Unhypnotized Subjects to Attitude Suggestions," ibid. 27 (July-August 1965):317-29.

27. Walter Cannon, *Bodily Changes in Pain, Hunger, Fear and Rage* (New York: Harper Torchback, 1963), pp. 355-56, 370.

28. Donald Hebb, *The Organization of Behavior: A Neurophysiological Theory* (New York: John Wiley and Sons, 1949), p. 237. At this point things get sticky. Hebb does not recognize that James rejected the Jacksonian contention that consciousness begins at a higher level. So Hebb is rejecting Cannon's critique of James on Cannon's own Jacksonian grounds.

James explained his theory to his friend Charles Renouvier as follows: "I don't mean that emotion is the perception of bodily changes *as such*, but only that bodily changes give us a feeling which is emotion. . . . After all, what my theory has in view is only the determination of the particular nerve process which emotion accompanies. We are bound to suppose that there is *some* such nerve process accompanying every emotion. Now all I say is that the nerve process is the incoming currents, produced by the reflex movements which the perception of the exciting cause engenders." James to Renouvier, September 30, 1884, in Perry, *The Thought and Character of William*

James, 2 vols. (Boston: Little, Brown and Co., 1935), 1:698.

29. Walter Cannon, dedication of *The Wisdom of the Body,* rev. ed. (New York: W. W. Norton, 1939). In his autobiographical, *The Way of an Investigator* (New York: W. W. Norton, 1945), pp. 19, 175, Cannon named Perry as one of his two closest friends. He also pointed out that at Harvard he had taken courses from James, considering him one of three professors who influenced him most.

30. Cannon, *Bodily Changes,* pp. 374-75.

31. Cannon, "New Evidence," pp. 26, 29.

32. In 1934, Cobb named Cannon one of the six major contributors to psychiatry in this century. Stanley Cobb, "Problems in Cerebral Anatomy and Physiology," in National Research Council, *The Problem of Mental Disorder* (New York, McGraw-Hill Book Co., 1934), pp. 111-19, 119.

33. Stanley Cobb, *Emotions and Clinical Medicine* (New York: W. W. Norton, 1950), pp. 65, 87.

34. John Fulton and C. F. Jacobsen, "The Functions of the Frontal Lobes, a Comparative Study in Monkeys, Chimpanzees and Man," *Abstracts from the Second International Neurological Congress* (London, Minor Publications, 1935), pp. 70-71.

35. John Fulton, *Frontal Lobotomy and Affective Behavior* (New York: W. W. Norton, 1951), pp. 17-18.

36. Freeman and Watts, *Psychosurgery,* pp. 399, 524, 538.

37. Ibid., pp. 386, 389-91.

38. Ibid., pp. 19, 237.

39. Ibid., pp. 407, 437-38.

40. Walter Freeman, *The Psychiatrist: Personalities and Patterns* (New York: Grune and Stratton, 1968), p. 137.

41. Freeman and Watts, *Psychosurgery,* p. 418.

42. Milton Greenblatt and Harry Solomon, "Concerning a Theory of Frontal Lobe Functioning," in *Frontal Lobes and Schizophrenia. Second Lobotomy Project at Boston Psychopathic Hospital,* eds. Greenblatt and Solomon (New York: Springer Publishing Co., 1953), pp. 408-10.

43. D. Levinson et al., "The Relation of Frontal Lobe Surgery to Intellectual and Emotional Functioning," in ibid., pp. 195-210.

44. Greenblatt and Solomon, "Concerning a Theory," p. 396.

45. Ibid., pp. 397-98.

46. Cobb, *Emotions and Clinical Medicine,* pp. 36-41.

47. G. Elliot Smith, *The Evolution of Man: Essays* (London: Oxford University Press, 1924), 30-33.

48. C. Judson Herrick, *Brains of Rats and Men* (New York: Hafner Publishing Co., 1963), pp. 134, 135, 232.

49. C. Judson Herrick, *The Thinking Machine* (Chicago: University of Chicago Press, 1929), p. 244.

50. H. Klüver and P. C. Bucy, "Preliminary Analysis of Functions of the Temporal Lobes in Monkeys," *Archives of Neurology and Psychiatry* 42 (December 1939):979-1000.

51. C. Judson Herrick, "Morphogenesis of the Brain," *Journal of Morphology* 54 (March 1933):233-58; "The Functions of the Olfactory Parts of the Cerebral Cortex," *Proceedings: National Academy of Sciences* 19 (January 1933):7-14.

52. James Papez, "A Proposed Mechanism of Emotion," *Archives of Neurology and Psychiatry* 38 (October 1937):743.

53. Paul MacLean, "Psychosomatic Disease and the 'Visceral Brain': Recent Developments on the Papez Theory of Emotion," *Psychosomatic Medicine* 11 (November-December 1949):338-53.

54. Paul MacLean, "The Limbic System ('Visceral Brain') in Relation to Central Gray and Reticulum of the Brain Stem," *Psychosomatic Medicine* 17 (September-October 1955):355-66; MacLean, "Contrasting Functions of Limbic and Neocortical Systems of the Brain and Their Relevance to Psychophysiological Aspects of Medicine," *The American Journal of Medicine* 25 (October 1958):611-26.

55. Paul MacLean, "Some Psychiatric Implications of Physiological Studies in Frontotemporal Portion of the Limbic System (Visceral Brain)," *Electroencephalography and Clinical Neurophysiology* 4 (November 1952):415.

56. Ibid., p. 414.

57. MacLean, "The Limbic System," p. 359.

58. MacLean, "Some Psychiatric Implications," p. 410.

CHAPTER 8. CONCEPTUAL LOBOTOMY

1. Karl Bowman and Milton Rose, "What is Schizophrenia?" in *Schizophrenia: An Integrated Approach,* ed., Alfred Auerback (New York: Ronald Press, 1959), pp. 3, 5.

2. William Pious, "A Hypothesis about the Nature of Schizophrenic Behavior," in ed. Arthur Burton, *Psychotheraphy of the Psychoses* (New York: Basic Books, 1961), p. 43.

3. Robert Gibson, in "Panel: Schizophrenia," in ed., Gene Usdin *Psychoneurosis and Schizophrenia,* p. 174.

4. Elvin Semrad, in ibid., p. 181.

5. Eugene Gendlin, "Research in Psychotherapy with Schizophrenic patients and the Nature of the 'Illness'," *American Journal of Psychotherapy* 20 (January 1966):10.

6. Karl Menninger, "Toward a Unified Concept of Mental Illness," in *A Psychiatrist's World*, ed. B. H. Hall (New York: Viking Press, 1959), p. 517.

7. Loren Mosher, "Evaluation of Psychosocial Treatments," in eds., Mosher and Gunderson *Psychotherapy of Schizophrenia*, pp. 254, 255.

8. Thomas Szasz, "The Problem of Psychiatric Nosology," *American Journal of Psychiatry* 114 (November 1957):405-13.

9. Julius Steinfeld, *A New Approach to Schizophrenia* (New York: Merlin Press, 1956), pp. 11, 13.

10. Stanley Lesse, "Psychotherapy Training Institutes and Current Realities," *American Journal of Psychotherapy* 20 (April 1956):303.

11. Gene Usdin, "Introduction," *Schizophrenia: Biological and Psychological Perspectives*, ed. Usdin (New York: Brunner/Mazel, 1975), pp. xvi, ix.

12. Jerome Frank, *Persuasion and Healing: A Comparative Study of Psychotherapy* (Baltimore, Johns Hopkins Press, 1961), pp. 13-14, 161, 20, 24.

13. Jules Masserman, *A Psychiatric Odyssey* (New York: Science House, 1971), pp. 522, 413.

14. Jules Masserman, *The Practice of Dynamic Psychiatry* (Philadelphia: W. B. Saunders, 1955), pp. 467, 466.

15. Masserman, *Odyssey*, pp. 180-96.

16. Walter Cannon, S. W. Britton, "Studies in the Conditions of Activity in Endocrine Glands: Pseudoaffective Medulleadrenal Secretion," *American Journal of Physiology* 72 (April 1925):284.

17. Walter Cannon, *Bodily Changes in Pain, Hunger, Fear, and Rage: An Account of Researches into the Function of Emotional Excitement*, 2d ed. (New York: Harper & Row, 1963), p. 225.

18. Walter Cannon, "Organization for Physiological Homeostasis," *Physiological Review* 9 (July 1929):425.

19. Cannon, *The Wisdom of the Body*, rev. ed. (New York: W. W. Norton, 1939) p. 20.

20. Ibid., pp. 300-303, 116.

21. Ibid., p. 258.

22. Other studies at Yale showed that stimulation of the amygdala can induce fear and rage responses: B. R. Kaada, P. Anderson, J. Jansen, "Stimulation of the Amygdaloid Nuclear Complex in Unanesthetized Cats," *Neurology* 4 (January 1954):48-64; H. Ursin and B. R. Kaada, "Functional Localization within the Amygdaloid Complex in the Cat," *EEG Clinical Neurophysiology* 12 (February 1960):1-20.

23. G. Moruzzi and H. W. Magoun, "Brain Stem Reticular Formation and Activation of the EEG," *EEG and Clinical Neurophysiology* 1 (November, 1949):455-509.

24. Donald Lindsley, "Emotion," in *Handbook of Experimental Psychology*, ed. S. S. Stevens (New York: John Wiley, 1951), pp. 504-16.

25. H. W. Magoun, *The Waking Brain*, 2d ed. (Springfield, Ill.: Charles C. Thomas, 1963), pp. 113-15, 20-22, has put together an extensive bibliography of works in neurophysiology dealing with feedback systems; but see, R. Hernandez-Peon, "Reticular Mechanisms of Sensory Control," in *Sensory Communications*, ed. W. Rosenblith (New York: John Wiley, 1961), pp. 497-520; H. H. Jasper et al., "Corticofugal Projections to the Brain Stem," *Archives of Neurology and Psychiatry* 67 (February 1952):155-66; K. E. Hagbarth and D. I. B. Kerr, "Central Influences on Spinal Afferent Conduction," *Journal of Neurophysiology* 17 (May 1954):295-307; and Magoun's own discussion, *Waking Brain*, pp. 14-16, 54ff, 101-6.

26. See, for example, F. A. Mettler, "Perceptual Capacity, Functions of the Corpus Striatum and Schizophrenia," *Psychiatric Quarterly* 29 (January 1955):89-111.

27. S. L. Sherwood, "Consciousness, Adaptive Behavior, and Schizophrenia," in *Schizophrenia, Somatic Aspects*, ed. D. Richter (New York: The Macmillan Co., 1957), pp. 131, 132.

28. Claude Shannon and Warren Weaver, *Mathematical Theory of Communication* (Urbana: University of Illinois Press, 1949). For discussion, see John Pierce, *Symbols, Signals and Noise: The Nature and Process of Communication* (New York: Harper Torchbook, 1961).

29. J. Y. Letvin et al., "What the Frog's Eye Tells the Frog's Brain (1959), in *Perceptual Processing*, ed. Peter Dodwell (New York: Appleton-Century-Crofts, 1971), pp. 305-26.

30. See, for example, P. H. Venables, "Input Dysfunction in Schizophrenia," *Progress in Experimental Personality Research* 1 (1964):1-47; Donald Broadbent, *Perception and Communication* (New York: Pergamon Press, 1966); Gerald Aronson, "Crucial Aspects of Therapeutic Intervention," in *Psychotherapy of Schizophrenia*, ed. Loren Mosher and John Gunderson (New York: J. Aronson, 1975), pp. 43-51; J. L. Reed, "Schizophrenia Thought Disorders: A Review and Hypothesis," *Comparative Psychiatry* 11 (September 1970):403-32; Thomas Freeman, John Cameron, and Andrew McGhie, *Chronic Schizophrenia* (New York: International Universities Press, 1958); William Lothrop, "A Critical Review of Research in the Conceptual Thinking in Schizophrenia," *JNMD* 132 (February 1961):118-26; R. W. Payne, "Cognitive Abnormalities," in *Handbook of Abnormal Psychology*, ed. Hans Eysenck (New York: Basic Books, 1961), pp. 193-261; Loren Chapman, "Distractibility in the Conceptual Performance of Schizophrenics," *Journal of Abnormal and Social Psychology* 53 (November 1956):286-91.

31. J. W. Lovett Doust, "Consciousness in Schizophrenia as a Function of

Peripheral Microcirculation," in *Physiological Correlates of Psychological Disorder*, ed. Robert Rossler and Norman Greenfield (Madison: University of Wisconsin Press, 1962), pp. 61–96.

32. Russell Monroe, *Episodic Behavioral Disorders: A Psychodynamic and Neurophysiological Analysis* (Cambridge, Mass.: Harvard University Press, 1970). See his bibliography for references to publications growing out of the Tulane project.

33. R. L. Isaacson, *The Limbic System* (New York: Plenum Press, 1974).

34. Split-brain research is reviewed by Michael Gazzaniga, *The Bisected Brain* (New York: Appleton-Century-Crofts, 1970).

35. For a review of the literature, see Morris Moscovitch, "Information Processing and the Cerebral Hemispheres," in *Handbook of Behavioral Neurobiology*, Vol. 2, *Neuropsychology*, ed. Michael Gazzaniga (New York and London: Plenum Books, 1979), pp. 379–446.

36. Michael Gazzaniga, Joseph Le Doux, and Donald Wilson, "Beyond Commissurotomy: Clues to Consciousness," in ibid., 543–53.

37. Julian Jaynes, *The Origin of Consciousness in the Breakdown of the Bicameral Mind* (Boston: Houghton Mifflin Co., 1976).

38. Alf Brodal, *Neurological Anatomy: in Relation to Clinical Medicine*, 2d ed. (New York: Oxford University Press, 1969), pp. 348, 603.

39. John Eccles, *The Understanding of the Brain* (New York: McGraw-Hill Publishing Co., 1973), p. 100.

40. For the history of systems theory, I have leaned heavily on Robert Lilienfeld's *The Rise of Systems Theory: An Ideological Analysis* (New York: John Wiley, 1978).

41. See John Kenneth Galbraith, *The New Industrial State* (Boston: Houghton Mifflin Co., 1971); Joseph Bensman and Arthur Vidich, *The New American Society* (Chicago: Quadrangle, 1971); David Bazelon, *Power in America—The Politics of the New Class* (New York: New American Library, 1967); Benjamin Kleinberg, *American Society in the Postindustrial Age* (Columbus, Ohio: Charles E. Merrill, 1973); Theodore Lowi, *The End of Liberalism—Ideology, Policy, and the Crisis of Public Authority* (New York: W. W. Norton, 1969).

42. See Lilienfeld, *Rise of Systems Theory;* William Gray, "History and Development of General Systems Theory," in *General Systems Theory and Psychiatry*, ed. Gray, Frederick Duhl, Nicholas Rizzo (Boston: Little, Brown and Co., 1969), pp. 7–32; Karl Menninger, with Martin Mayman and Paul Pruyser, *The Vital Balance: The Life Process in Mental Health and Illness* (New York: The Viking Press, 1963), pp. 76–124.

43. See also Colin Cherry's *On Human Communication*, 2d ed. (Cambridge: MIT Press, 1978); Walter Fuch, *Computers—Information Theory and*

Cybernetics (London: Rupert Hart-Davis, 1971); Jagjit Singh, *Great Ideas in Information Theory, Language and Cybernetics* (New York: Dover, 1966); Donald MacKay, *Information, Mechanism, and Meaning* (Cambridge: MIT Press, 1969).

44. See Margaret Boden, *Artificial Intelligence and Natural Man* (New York: Basic Books, Inc., 1977); M. A. Arbib, *The Metaphorical Brain* (New York: Wiley-Interscience, 1972).

45. Jacques Monod, *Chance and Necessity* (New York: Alfred Knopf, 1971); Gregory Bateson, *Mind and Nature: A Necessary Unity* (New York: E. P. Dutton, 1979).

46. Gordon Allport, "The Open System in Personality Theory," *Journal of Abnormal and Social Psychology* 61 (November 1960):301-10.

47. See, for example, G. A. Miller, Eugene Galanter, and Karl Bribram, *Plans and the Structure of Behavior* (New York: Holt, Rinehart and Winston, 1960); Ulric Neisser, *Cognitive Psychology* (New York: Appleton-Century-Crofts, 1969); Walter Reitman, *Cognition and Thought: An Information Processing Approach* (New York: John Wiley, 1965); Peter Lindsay and Donald Norman, *Human Information Processing: An Introduction to Psychology* (New York: Academic Press, 1972); John Anderson and Gordon Bower, *Human Associative Memory* (Washington: V. H. Winston, 1973); G. A. Miller and P. N. Johnson-Laird, *Language and Perception* (Cambridge, Mass: Belknap Press, 1976); Allan Newell and Herbert Simon, *Human Problem Solving* (Englewood Cliffs, N.J.: Prentice-Hall, 1972); Donald Norman and D. E. Rumelhart, *Explorations in Cognition* (San Francisco: W. H. Freeman, 1975).

48. Ludwig von Bertalanffy, "General Systems Theory and Psychiatry—An Overview" (1967), in William Gray et al. eds., *General Systems Theory*, p. 40.

49. Warren McCulloch and Walter Pitts, "A Logical Calculus of Ideas Imminent in Nervous Activity" (1943), in McCulloch, *Embodiments of Mind* (Cambridge, Mass.: MIT Press, 1965), pp. 19-39.

50. Warren McCulloch, "Finality and Form," in ibid., pp. 256-75.

51. Bateson, *Mind and Nature*, pp. 58-59.

52. Menninger, *Vital Balance*, pp. 109, 114ff.

53. See Robert Powell, "Helen Flanders Dunbar (1902-1959) and a Holistic Approach to Psychosomatic Problems. I. The Rise and Fall of a Medical Philosophy," *Psychiatric Quarterly* 49 (Summer 1977):133-52.

54. William Gray and Nicholas Rizzo, "History and Development of General Systems Theory," in Gray et al., *General Systems Theory*, p. 17.

55. Roy Grinker, "Comparisons Between Systems of Organization," in *Toward a Unified Theory of Human Behavior*, ed. Grinker, (New York: Basic Books, Inc., 1956), p. 137.

56. James Toman, "Multiple Origins of the Uniqueness of Human Society," in ibid., pp. 145, 146.

57. Lawrence Frank, "Social Systems and Culture," in ibid., p. 204.

58. Grinker, "Comparison Between Systems," p. 139.

59. Edgar Auerswald, "Interdisciplinary Versus Ecological Approach," in Gray et al., *General Systems Theory*, pp. 373-86.

60. Don Jackson, "The Individual and the Larger Contexts," in ibid., p. 388.

BIBLIOGRAPHICAL ESSAY

MANUSCRIPTS.

The William James papers at the Houghton Library, Harvard University, are invaluable, although much of his correspondence and parts of his diary can be found in publications, such as Ralph Barton Perry's two volume classic, *The Thought and Character of William James* (Boston: Little, Brown and Co., 1935); *The Letters of William James*, 2 vols., ed. Henry James (Boston: The Atlantic Monthly Press, 1920); *The Letters of William James and Theodore Flournoy*, ed. Robert Le Clair (Madison: University of Wisconsin Press, 1966). The papers of G. Stanley Hall, such as they are, are at Clark University. They give important insights into his youthful thinking and contain some unpublished speeches. Adolf Meyer's correspondence and case histories will provide a gold mine for historians in the future, but they are still uncatalogued at Johns Hopkins University. William Alanson White's papers for his long years at St. Elizabeth's are complete at the National Archives. James Jackson Putnam's papers, at the Francis A. Countway Library of Medicine in Boston, are to be supplemented by Nathan Hale, *James Jackson Putnam and Psychoanalysis: Letters Between Putnam and Sigmund Freud, Ernest Jones, William James, Sandor Ferenci and Morton Prince, 1877-1917* (Cambridge, Mass.: Harvard University Press, 1971). Some of Harry Stack Sullivan's correspondence, especially with White, is collected at the William Alanson White Foundation, Washington, D.C.

GENERAL.

My debt to George Herbert Mead (*Mind, Self, and Society*, Chicago: University of Chicago Press, 1934) has already been expressed, as has my debt to Max Horkheimer, *Eclipse of Reason*, (New York: The Seabury Press, 1974); *Critique of Instrumental Reason*, trans. Matthew O'Connell (New York: Seabury Press, 1974); Theodor Adorno et al., *The Authoritarian Personality* (New York: Harper and Row, Publishers, 1950); and Herbert Marcuse,

Reason and Revolution: Hegel and the Rise of Social Theory, 2d ed. (Boston: Beacon Press, 1964); *One-Dimensional Man: Studies in the Ideology of Advanced Industrial Society* (Boston: Beacon Press, 1964). My reliance on David Riesman, *The Lonely Crowd: A Study of the Changing American Character* (New Haven: Yale University Press, 1950) is, no doubt, everywhere evident.

Several excellent studies helped me get at the doxological mapping in the biological sciences that preceded the Darwinian revolution. Margaret Jacob's *The Newtonians and the English Revolution* (Ithaca: Cornell University Press, 1976) is excellent on the class balance to which the Newtonian synthesis spoke. This is in contrast with earlier class theorizing inaugurated by Robert Merton's "Science, Technology, and Society in Seventeenth Century England," *Orisis* 4 (1938):360-632. For another balanced view, see Charles Webster's *The Great Instauration: Science, Medicine and Reform, 1626-1660* (New York: Holmes and Meier, Publishers, 1975). In her *Man and Society: The Scottish Inquiry of the Eighteenth Century* (Princeton: Princeton University Press, 1945), Gladys Bryson forcefully pointed out the importance of Newtonian science with its ordering of the phenomenal realm for the Scottish commonsense philosophers. Adam Smith, for example, believed that "Philosophy, by representing the invisible chains which bind together all those disjointed objects [of experience], endeavors to induce order into this chaos of jarring and discordant appearances" (p. 16). The spirit of the doxological science in America is captured by Theodore Dwight Bozeman, *Protestants in an Age of Science: The Baconian Ideal and Antebellum Religious Thought* (Chapel Hill: University of North Carolina Press, 1977), and by George Daniels, *American Science in the Age of Jackson* (New York: Columbia University Press, 1968). However, to get at the resistance to the mechanistic cause-effect scheme in the pre-Darwinian biological sciences, it is necessary to go back to the sources. Daniel Boorstin, *The Lost World of Thomas Jefferson* (New York: Henry Holt and Co., 1948) defines the functionalist rationale that crept into the deepest recesses of the American Enlightenment.

Beginning with Marvin Meyers, *The Jacksonian Persuasion: Politics and Belief* (Stanford: Stanford University Press, 1957), the trend in the historical study of the Jacksonian period has been toward seeing the age through the eyes of de Tocqueville, as a period marked by the absence of class and institutional structure and because of this absence, suffused with anxiety. Winthrop Jordan's *White Over Black* (Baltimore: Penguin Books, 1969) was a major force in beginning the psychological investigation of the period with the absence of strong social structure as the starting point, although Stanley Elkins's *Slavery: A Problem in American Institutional Life* (Chicago: University of Chicago Press, 1959), which deals with slave psychology, preceded it.

The psychological theorizing based on the concept of the effects of a too-loosely structured society has been introduced into medicine and psychiatry by G. J. Barker-Benfield's *Horrors of the Half-Known Life: Male Attitudes toward Women and Sexuality in Nineteenth-Century America* (New York: Harper and Row, Publishers, 1976), which is suggestive, but Freudian, and David Rothman's *The Discovery of the Asylum: Social Order and Disorder in the New Republic* (Boston: Little, Brown and Co., 1971).

Concerning the underside of the Victorian mind in literature, besides Kenneth Lynn's *William Dean Howells: An American Life* (New York: Harcourt, Brace, Jovanovich, 1970, 1971), which does an excellent job of getting into the genteel family, see Harry Levin, *The Power of Blackness: Hawthorne, Poe, Melville* (New York: Alfred Knopf, Publisher, 1958). In the area of medicine, John and Robin Haller's *The Physician and Sexuality in Victorian America* (New York: W. W. Norton and Co., 1977) contains suggestive material. Still in the general area of medicine, Michel Foucault's *Madness and Civilization: A History of Insanity in the Age of Reason*, trans. Richard Howard, (New York: Pantheon Books, 1968) lays a broad basis for the understanding of nineteenth-century perceptions of insanity. His thesis concerns the loss of the "dialogue" between "reason" and "unreason" during the seventeenth and eighteenth centuries. Exactly what he means by these terms is never quite clear to me, but his "unreason" is obviously something of the nature of what I call the Victorian "underside," but seen as a kind of force or voice in its own right and with a logic of its own. From my Jamesian angle, which interprets the "unconscious" as the "fringe" and "subliminal" (that is, an opening out to the ineffable), French structuralism seems plagued by assumptions I have attempted to critique throughout the book. To my mind, similar objections can be brought against the otherwise brilliant work of Erich Kahler, *Man the Measure* (New York: George Braziller, 1943); *The Tower and the Abyss: An Inquiry into the Transformation of the Individual* (New York: George Braziller, 1957), whose theme is the juxtaposition of community and the collective.

For my understanding of the nature of traditional society, especially the function of ceremony, I have relied on the work of Mircea Eliade (for example, *The Sacred and the Profane*, trans. Willard Trask (New York: Harcourt, Brace and Co., 1959). The work of Philip Aries, in his *Centuries of Childhood: A Social History of Family Life*, trans. Robert Baldick (New York: Alfred Knopf, Publisher, 1962) ties the emerging privacy of family life to the rise of the middle class and has large implications for the nineteenth-century middle-class family's adjustment to the capitalist marketplace. Peter Berger, Brigitte Berger, and Hansfried Kellner's, *The Homeless Mind: Modernization of Consciousness* (New York: Random House, 1973) speaks somewhat to this question, but it is not as powerful as its title suggests. The question of privacy of experiencing is explored in several works on seventeenth-century autobiographical writings. Owen Watkins, *The Puritan Experience: Studies in Spiritual Autobiography* (New York: Schocken Books, 1972) argues for a "growing self-consciousness" due to increasing complexity of society and culture, and an extreme sense of alienation from God. Paul Delany, *British Autobiography in the Seventeenth Century* (London: Routledge and Kegan Paul, 1969) asserts that personal identity was unprecedently elusive. John Morris's *Versions of the Self: Studies in English Autobiography from John Bunyon to John Stuart Mill* (New York: Basic Books, 1966) makes the same kinds of points. It is time for a study of the seventeenth-century scientific revolution in the context of its attempt to restore the public reality in face of this growing privacy of experiencing. Christopher Lasch, *The New Radicalism in America, 1889-1963* (New York: Vintage Books, 1965) takes the children of the genteel and skillfully develops their personal motives for going into reform. He develops many of the themes I have touched on and, in the process, manages to be both broad and deep. On the sexual side of the Victorian underside, see Steven Marcus, *The Other Victorians: A Study of Sexuality and Pornography in Mid-Nineteenth Century England* (New York: Basic Books, 1964).

Historians of the rise of the mechanistic philosophy have yet to delve deeply into the distinction between an atomism of order and an atomism of random flux. Edwin Burtt's classic, *The Metaphysical Foundations of Modern Physical Science* (London: Kegan Paul, Trench, Trubner and Co., 1925) laid the foundation for such an approach, but there has been little follow-up. See Maria Boas, "The Establishment of the Mechanical Philosophy," *Orisis* 10 (1952):412-541; E. J. Dijksterhuis, *The Mechanization of the World Picture*, trans. C. Dikshoorn (Oxford: Clarendon Press, 1961); Robert Schofield, *Mechanism and Materialism: British Natural Philosophy in an Age of Reason* (Princeton: Princeton University Press, 1970); Joshua Gregory, *A Short History of Atomism* (London: A. and C. Black, 1931). On Locke's atomism, see Maurice Mandelbaum, *Philosophy, Science, and Sense Perception* (Baltimore: Johns Hopkins Press, 1964). For specialized studies in the nineteenth century, see Wilson Scott, *The Conflict Between Atomism and Conservation Theory, 1644-1860* (London: Macdonald and Co., 1970), and *The Atomic Debates*, ed. William Brock (Leicester: Leicester University Press, 1967). But the grandest of all studies concerning the mechanical philosophy is Ernst Cassirer, *The Philosophy of the Enlightenment*, trans. Fritz Koelin and James Pettegrove, (Princeton: Princeton University Press, 1951).

Finally, I should make clear my debt to two general works on the nature of science: Thomas Kuhn, *The Structure of Scientific Revolutions*, 2d ed. (Chicago:

University of Chicago Press, 1970), who has done for the understanding of science what Edward Sapir did for language; and Charles Gillispie, *The Edge of Objectivity: An Essay in the History of Scientific Ideas* (Princeton: Princeton University Press, 1960), who so beautifully expressed the scientific faith against which I am reacting.

CHAPTER 1. SELFHOOD AND INSANITY

The studies of nineteenth-century medicine and neuropsychiatry are numerous, excellent, and form an essential background for understanding the movements I have discussed. First, in order of precedence, stands the work of Richard Shryock, *Medicine and Society in America, 1660-1860* (Ithaca: Cornell University Press, 1960), and *The Development of Modern Medicine: An Interpretation of the Social and Scientific Factors Involved* (New York: Hafner Publishing Co., 1969). Three studies form the backbone for all further work in nineteenth-century American psychiatry: Albert Deutsch, *The Mentally Ill in America*, 2d rev. ed. (New York: Columbia University Press, 1949); Gerald Grob, *The State and the Mentally Ill* (Chapel Hill: University of North Carolina Press, 1966); and Norman Dain, *Concepts of Insanity in the United States, 1789-1863* (New Brunswick: Rutgers University Press, 1964). Close upon these, but somewhat more specialized, are: Charles Rosenberg, *The Trial of the Assassin Guiteau* (Chicago: University of Chicago Press, 1968), John Davies, *Phrenology, Fad and Science: A 19th Century Crusade* (New Haven: Yale University Press, 1955); Arthur Fink, *Causes of Crime: Biological Theories in the United States* (Philadelphia: University of Pennsylvania Press, 1938), and Mark Haller, *Eugenics: Hereditarian Attitudes in American Thought* (New Brunswick: Rutgers University Press, 1963). Ruth Caplan's *Psychiatry and Community in Nineteenth Century America* (New York: Basic Books, 1969) should also be consulted. Indispensable works that are more general in nature are George Rosen, *Madness and Society: Chapters in the Historical Sociology of Mental Illness* (London: Routledge and Kegan Paul, 1968); Henri Ellenberger, *The Discovery of the Unconscious* (New York: Basic Books, 1970); Franz Alexander and Sheldon Selesnick, *The History of Psychiatry* (New York: Harper and Row, Publishers, 1966); Edwin Boring, *A History of Experimental Psychology*, 2d ed. (New York: Appleton, Century, Crofts, 1950); Gregory Zilboorg and George Henry, *History of Medical Psychology* (Philadelphia: J. B. Lippincott, 1954). The trend of these general studies is pre-Kuhn, in the sense that they take the position that science is a steady advance out of the darkness into the light.

More specific studies that speak to important aspects of my story are: E. T. Carlson, "The Influence of Phrenology on Early American Psychiatric Thought,"

American Journal of Psychiatry 115 (December 1958):535-38; June Goodfield, *The Growth of Scientific Physiology: Physiological Method and the Mechanist-Vitalist Controversy* (New York: Arno Press, 1975); Eric Carlson and Norman Dain, "The Meaning of Moral Insanity," *Bulletin of the History of Medicine* 36 (March-April 1962):130-40; Owsei Temkin, *The Falling Sickness: A History of Epilepsy from the Greeks to the Beginnings of Modern Neurology* (Baltimore: Johns Hopkins Press, 1945). Temkin gets importantly into the work of John Hughlings Jackson and in many ways is reinforced by Robert Young's *Mind, Brain and Adaptation in the Nineteenth Century: Cerebral Localization and its Biological Context from Gall to Ferrier* (Oxford: Clarendon Press, 1970). Perhaps this is the place to reiterate my own position. Young holds that by following Spencer and bringing Darwinian evolution into neurophysiology, Hughlings Jackson not only established the modern structure for neurophysiology but revivified the idea that I have been calling the higher-lower doctrine. My feeling is that the doctrine was very much alive without Darwinian evolution, and that it absorbed the evolutionary idea into it and made it work for it. The backbone of the higher-lower doctrine was not the evolutionary theory, or even Jackson's level theory, it was the perceptual processes of the psychiatrists and neurologists.

The best work on S. Weir Mitchell is still Anna Robeson Burr, *Weir Mitchell. His Life and Letters* (New York: Duffield, 1930). For George Beard, see George Rosenberg, "The Place of George M. Beard in Nineteenth Century American Psychiatry," *Bulletin of the History of Medicine* 36 (May-June 1962):245-59. The biographer of Isaac Ray is Jacques Quen. See his "Isaac Ray and His 'Remarks on Pathological Anatomy,'" *Bulletin of the History of Medicine* 38 (March-April 1964):113-26; see also Winfred Overholzer's "Editor's Introduction," to Isaac Ray's *A Treatise on the Medical Jurisprudence of Insanity* (Boston: C. C. Little and J. Brown, 1838). Unfortunately, John P. Gray has not found his biographer, and one must be content with passing references in the histories, particularly Rosenberg's *Trial of the Assassin Guiteau*, Dain's *Concepts of Insanity*, and Grob's *State and the Mentally Ill.*

On the development of the mechanistic picture of nervous and mental action, see Young, *Mind, Brain and Adaptation;* Frederick Albert Lange, *The History of Materialism*, trans. Ernest Thomas (New York: The Humanities Press, 1925); Edward Liddell, *The Discovery of Reflexes* (Oxford: Clarendon Press, 1960); and several of the papers from *The History and Philosophy of Knowledge of the Brain and Its Functions*, ed. Frederick Poynter. Edwin Boring's work on the subject in his *History of Experimental Psychology* (New York: D. Appleton-Century Co., 1929) is a classic.

CHAPTER 2. IN SEARCH OF THE REAL MISS BEAUCHAMP

For an overview of Morton Prince and his colleagues, see Chapter 6 of Nathan Hale's *Freud and the Americans: The Beginnings of Psychoanalysis in the United States, 1876-1917* (New York: Oxford University Press, 1971). See also William Taylor, *Morton Prince and Abnormal Psychology* (New York: D. Appleton and Co., 1928). On Miss Beauchamp, see Otto Marx, "Morton Prince and the Dissociation of a Personality," *Journal of the History of the Behavioral Sciences* 6 (April 1970):120-30. See the historical summary of multiple personality cases by W. S. Taylor and M. F. Martin, "Multiple Personality," *Journal of Abnormal and Social Psychology* 39 (July 1944): 281-300. So far as I know, doubts about multiple personality have until now been limited to stressing the possibility that the "alternate personalities" were artifacts of hypnosis. For the European scene Ellenberger's *Discovery of the Unconscious* is best, but see also Georges Guillain's *J.-M. Charcot, 1825-1893: His Life, His Work* (Paris: Masson, 1955). Carol Smith and Charles Rosenberg's "The Female Animal: Medical and Biological Views of Woman and her Role in Nineteenth-Century America," *Journal of American History* 60 (September 1973):332-56, delves into the genteel reaction to the new freedoms women were beginning to feel and explore.

CHAPTER 3. VOICE FROM THE ABYSS: WILLIAM JAMES

Everything since Ralph Barton Perry's *The Thought and Character of William James*, 2 vols. (Boston: Little, Brown and Co., 1935) has been a footnote to that work. Gay Wilson Allen's major biography, *William James: A Biography* (New York: The Viking Press, 1967) corrects Perry's tendency to emphasize James's healthy-mindedness, as does the work Leon Edel has been doing on brother Henry. Other than the two biographies mentioned, most of the work on James has been either critique or classification. Two major areas of James's life and work need to be developed, it seems to me: on one side, his work in parapsychology needs to be taken more seriously (for example, see Gardner Murphy and Robert Ballou, eds. *William James on Psychical Research*, [New York: The Viking Press, 1960]) as central to his thinking about abnormal mental states and religious experience, with the end in view of integrating it into (and hence broadening out) his philosophy. On the other side, his attitudes toward and conception of evil needs a thorough examination in order to develop a firmer understanding of his philosophy of freedom and possibility. Both these areas of research have been blocked, I assume, by the tendency to overemphasize James's sunny side.

One of the more confusing aspects of James's philosophy is his notion of chance. Edward Madden's *Chauncey Wright and the Foundations of Pragmatism* (Seattle: University of Washington Press, 1963) is extremely helpful in making the distinction between the apparent chance Wright embraced and the absolute chance defined by Charles S. Peirce and picked up by James.

CHAPTER 4. COMMUNITY: APOTHEOSIS OF THE REAL MISS BEAUCHAMP

Dorothy Ross's *G. Stanley Hall: The Psychologist as Prophet* (Chicago: University of Chicago Press, 1972) is excellent, and replaces Lorine Pruett's *G. Stanley Hall: A Biography of Mind* (New York: D. Appleton and Co., 1926) as the standard. Both are to be supplemented by the sections on Hall in R. Jackson Wilson's *In Quest of Community: Social Philosophy in the United States, 1860-1920* (New York: John Wiley and Sons, 1968), and Charles Strickland and Charles Burges, *Health, Growth and Heredity: G. Stanley Hall on Natural Education* (New York: Teachers College Press, 1965), Boring's *History of Experimental Psychology*, and John Winkler and Walter Bromberg's *Mind Explorers* (New York: Reynal and Hitchcock, 1939). See also Hall's own *Life and Confessions of a Psychologist* (New York: D. Appleton and Co., 1932), and his "Note on Early Memories," in *Recreations of a Psychologist* (New York: D. Appleton and Co., 1920). For insight into Hall's reaction to Freud, see John Burnham, "Sigmund Freud and G. Stanley Hall: Exchange of Letters," *Psychoanalytic Quarterly* 29 (July 1960):307-16.

I know of no studies on the psychology of religion movement. Frank Manuel's *The Eighteenth Century Confronts the Gods* (Cambridge, Mass.: Harvard University Press, 1959) was more helpful than the one or two formal histories of anthropology.

On the New Realism, see the short and precise discussion by Morris Cohen, *American Thought, A Critical Sketch* (Glencoe, Ill.: Free Press, 1954), and the longer and more thorough one by William Werkmeister, in *A History of Philosophical Ideas in America* (New York: Ronald Press Co., 1948), which treats the New Realists as rebels against the idealism of Josiah Royce. The appearance of the New Realism brought forth an immediate burst of criticism. See, for example, Morris Cohen, "The New Realism," *Journal of Philosophy* 10 (April 10, 1913):197-214; E. H. Holland's attack on the New Realist doctrine of "The Externality of Relations," *Journal of Philosophy* 11 (August 13, 1914):463-69, and the emergence (in reaction) of an even newer school (Critical Realism) in, for example, Arthur O. Lovejoy's "Realism versus Epistemological Monism," *Journal of Philosophy* 10 (October 9, 1913):561-71. A blow-by-blow account with bibliography of the New Realism, the Critical Realist reaction, and then the stabilization of the monistic position in the work of philosophers like Whitehead is given in Victor Harlow, *A Bibliography and Genetic Study of American Realism* (New York: Kraus Reprint, 1970).

CHAPTER 5. THE AMERICANIZATION OF FREUDIANISM AND SCHIZOPHRENIA

The material on Freud is voluminous; I have cited some of it in footnotes to chapter 5. Freud sometimes made it clear that the unconscious is not to be considered an entity. It is a group of processes. But Freud also visualized those processes within the higher-lower doctrine and multiple personality contexts, and in those contexts, it emerged as an entity or even a self. All the authors whom I have encountered assumed the reality of the unconscious and saw Freud as its great explorer. This is true even of Lancelot Whyte, *The Unconscious before Freud* (New York: Basic Books, 1960), whose insightful discussion of self-consciousness is, to my mind, thereby distorted or even negated. For the same reason, the mental health liberal's ideal community and the Real Miss Beauchamp should not be confused with the "therapeutic society" and "psychological man" pictured by Philip Rieff in *Freud: The Mind of the Moralist*, 3d ed. (Chicago: University of Chicago Press, 1979).

The importance of Hughlings Jackson for Freud has been gaining recognition since the work of Erwin Stengel (for example, "The Origins and Status of Dynamic Psychology," *British Journal of Medical Psychology* 27 [Part 4, 1954]:193–200), as may be seen in Frank Sulloway, *Freud, Biologist of the Mind* (New York: Basic Books, 1979) and other works cited in chapter 5 footnotes. But the recognition has not, as I believe it must, turned historians' attention to the profound effect on psychoanalytic theory of English anthropology and its notions of the primitive mind.

The Americanization of Freudian theory has received a good amount of thoughtful analysis. John Burnham's *Psychoanalysis and American Medicine, 1894–1918. Medicine, Science and Culture*, vol. 4, *Psychological Issues* (New York: International Universities Press, 1967) argues that Freudianism was less esteemed in America for its specific doctrines than for the support it seemed to give to beliefs in evolution, psychotherapy, and progressive reform. My point, that Freudianism was seen as a support for the higher-lower doctrine is, in a sense, a refinement on Burnham's theme. But my thesis that American Freudianism was part of a reaction against the breakdown of nineteenth-century controls contrasts with the position taken by Nathan Hale (*Freud and the Americans: The Beginnings of Psychoanalysis in the United States, 1876–1917* [New York: Oxford University Press, 1971]) that American Freudianism was a rebellion against Victorian self-control and repression. One should also consult John Seeley's *The Americanization of the Unconscious* (New York: International Universities Press, 1967).

In his "From Berggasse XIX to Central Park West: The Americanization of Psychoanalysis, 1918-1940," *Journal of the History of the Behavioral Sciences* 14 (October 1978):299-315, Nathan Hale describes the growth of a professional medical elite and its emphasis on individual adjustment. It was probably Roy Lubove (*The Professional Altruist: The Emergence of Social Work as a Career, 1880-1930* [New York: Harvard University Press, 1965]) who first successfully brought together the themes of professionalization, psychotherapy, and social control through emphasis on personal adjustment. These themes are renewed in F. H. Matthews, "The Americanization of Sigmund Freud: Adaptations of Psychoanalysis before 1917," *Journal of American Studies* 1 (April 1967):39-62, and by John Burnham's "The New Psychology: From Narcissism to Social Control," in *Change and Continuity in Twentieth Century America: The 1920's*, ed. John Braeman, Robert Bremner, David Brody (Columbus: Ohio State University Press, 1968) pp. 351-98. In his "From Avant-Garde to Specialism: Psychoanalysis in America," *Journal of the History of the Behavioral Sciences* 15 (April, 1979):128-34, John Burnham balanced the picture by describing the psychoanalysts as bearers of humanitarianism and rationalism.

See Nathan Hale's biographical essay on Putnam in his *James Jackson Putnam and Psychoanalysis: Letters Between Putnam and Sigmund Freud, Ernest Jones, William James, Sandor Ferenczi, and Morton Prince, 1877-1917* (Cambridge: Harvard University Press, 1971) and his discussion of Putnam in *Freud and the Americans*. See Karl Menninger's "Smith Ely Jelliffe," in his *A Psychiatrist's World*, and for White see the essays in *William Alanson White: The Washington Years, 1903-1937*, ed. Arcangelo D'Amore (Washington, D.C.: U.S. Department of Health, Education and Welfare, 1976), as well as White's own autobiographical efforts: *Forty Years of Psychiatry* (New York and Washington: Journal of Nervous and Mental Disease Publishing Co., 1933), and *William Alanson White: The Autobiography of a Purpose* (Garden City, N.Y.: Doubleday, Doran, 1938). There is some autobiographical material in *Edward J. Kempf: Selected Papers*, ed. Dorothy Clarke Kempf and John Burnham, (Bloomington, Ind.: Indiana University Press, 1974). For Adolf Meyer, see Hale's *Freud and the Americans* and Burnham's *Psychoanalysis and American Medicine* for short discussions, and Alfred Lief's *The Commonsense Psychiatry of Dr. Adolf Meyer* (New York: McGraw-Hill Publishing Co., 1948) for a more personalized account, which, however, is a bit rambling. See also, Eunice Winters, "Adolf Meyer's Two and a Half Years at Kankakee," *Bulletin of the History of Medicine* 40 (September-October 1966):441-58.

Clarence Oberndorf's *A History of Psychoanalysis in America* (New York: Grune and Stratton, 1953) takes us inside the fledgling orthodox psychoanalytic movement of the early years.

CHAPTER 6. PSYCHIATRY: A FADING SCIENCE

A. H. Chapman's *Harry Stack Sullivan: His Life and Work* (New York: G. P. Putnam, 1976), correctly, I believe, takes Sullivan out of the "neo-Freudian" category where he is usually put (for example, in Dieter Wyss, *Depth Psychology: A Critical History, Development, Problems, Crises* (New York: W. W. Norton, 1966). But because of the absolute dearth of sources, Chapman's book is but a small advance on what we already know about Sullivan's life from Helen Swick Perry's "Introduction," to Sullivan, *Personal Psychopathology* (New York: W. W. Norton and Co., 1965), her "Introduction" to Harry Stack Sullivan, *Schizophrenia as a Human Process* (New York: W. W. Norton and Co., 1962), and Clara Thompson's "Harry Stack Sullivan, the Man," in Sullivan, *Schizophrenia as a Human Process*. Walter Freeman's comments on Sullivan in *The Psychiatrist: Personalities and Patterns* (New York: Grune and Stratton, 1968) are motivated by antipathy.

Thomas Szasz has done yeoman work in developing a critique of recent American psychiatry (for example, *The Myth of Mental Illness: Foundations of a Theory of Personal Conduct* [London: Secker and Warburg, 1961]; *The Manufacture of Madness: A Comparative Study of the Inquisition and Mental Health* [New York: Harper and Row, 1970]), thus making it easier for the historian to take a post-Kuhnian view of the subject. However, the blanket assertion that mental illness is simply a label for social deviance has the unfortunate effect of shifting the focus away from historical developments. The same kind of thing can be said for popularizers of the Szasz approach (for example, Ronald Leifer, *In the Name of Mental Health: The Social Functions of Psychiatry* [New York: Science House, 1969]). Maurice North's *The Secular Priests* (London: Allen and Unwin, 1972), which implicates psychiatry as part of the service oriented bureaucracy doing work for the technological society, has much to recommend it.

CHAPTER 7. PSYCHOSURGERY: SCIENCE CONFRONTS THE BIZARRE

Outright critical studies and accounts of the inner history of psychosurgery are nonexistent. But there are any number of studies done within the profession of neurophysiology on the fruits (or lack thereof) of the psychosurgical process. See, for example: Manuel Riklan and Eric Levita, *Subcortical Corre-*

lates of Human Behavior: A Psychological Study of Thalamic and Basal Ganglia Surgery (Baltimore: Williams and Wilkins Co., 1969); Lothar Kalinowsky and Paul Hoch, *Shock Treatments, Psychosurgery and other Somatic Treatments in Psychiatry,* 2d ed. (New York: Grune and Stratton, 1952); G. K. Yacorzynski, Benjamin Boshes, and Loyal Davis, "Psychological Changes Produced by Frontal Lobotomy," in Association for Research in Nervous and Mental Disease, *The Frontal Lobes,* vol. 27, *Research Publications* (Baltimore: Williams and Wilkins Co., 1948); Jan Frank, "Clinical Survey and Results of 200 Cases of Profrontal Leucotomy," *Journal of Mental Science* 92 (July 1946):497-508.

Most accounts of twentieth-century American neurophysiology are textbook-style summaries of major stages of development. However, see Nigel Calder, *The Mind of Man: An Investigation into Current Research on the Brain and Human Nature* (New York: Viking Press, 1970), and Daniel Robinson, *The Enlightened Machine: An Analytical Introduction to Neurophysiology* (Encino, Calif.: Dickinson Publications, 1973). For personal accounts of the group of investigations following up the Magoun-Moruzzi reticular formation breakthrough, see Frederic Worden, Judith Swazey, and George Adelman, eds., *The Neurosciences: Paths of Discovery* (Cambridge, Mass.: MIT Press, 1975).

CHAPTER 8. CONCEPTUAL LOBOTOMY

The material on one or another of the aspects of systems theory is now endless. In addition to material in the footnotes, the following is suggested. For information theory in neurophysiology, see Lila Gatlin, *Information Theory and the Living System* (New York: Columbia University Press, 1972); *Information Storage and Neural Control,* ed. W. S. Fields and Walter Abbott (Springfield, Ill.: Charles C. Thomas, 1963). The related field of cybernetics is perhaps best described by its inventor, Norbert Wiener (for example, *Cybernetics, or, Control and Communication in the Animal and Machine* [Cambridge, Mass.: MIT Press, 1948]). And the attempt to bring systems theory into biology is illustrated in Ludwig von Bertalanffy, *Problems of Life, An Evaluation of Modern Biological Thought* (New York: John Wiley, 1952). The parallel attempt to bring it into the behavioral sciences is seen in Walter Buckley, ed., *Modern Systems Research for the Behavioral Sciences* (Chicago: Aldine Publishing Co., 1968), and into philosophy in Ervin Laszlo, *System, Structure and Experience: Toward a Scientific Theory of Mind* (New York: Gordon and Breach, 1968), and Ervin Laszlo, *The Systems View of the World: The Natural Philosophy of the New Developments in the Sciences* (New York: George Braziller, 1972).

Much of the controversy surrounding systems theory centers on the idea of artificial intelligence, the notion that the computer is an adequate model for the brain. Two introductory books are: Michael Arbib, *The Metaphorical Brain* (New York: Wiley-Interscience, 1972), and F. H. George, *The Brain as a Computer* (Oxford: Pergamon Press, 1962). One of the central problems of this assertion revolves around the uses and powers of formal logic. An introduction is Michael Arbib, *Brains, Machines, and Mathematics* (New York: McGraw-Hill, 1964). Asking what the limits of the computer are involves delving into the limits of mathematical logic, for example, Ernest Nagel and James Newman, *Gödel's Proof* (New York: New York University Press, 1960); Neil Jones, *Computability Theory: An Introduction* (New York: Academic Press, 1973); Martin Davis, *Computability and Unsolvability* (New York: McGraw-Hill Publishing Co., 1958). And lest one think that the questions involved are sterile, one should take a look at Douglas Hofstadter's *Gödel, Escher, Bach: An Eternal Golden Braid* (New York: Basic Books, Inc., 1979).

INDEX

About the Author

S. P. FULLINWIDER is Associate Professor of History at Arizona State University in Tempe and the author of *The Mind and Mood of Black America* among other publications.